Suffer
The Little
Children

Suffer
The Little
Children

the battle
against childhood cancer

by Dr. Jocelyn Demers
with a preface by Dr. Stuart Siegel

translated by James Parry

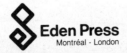

Eden Press
Montréal - London

Suffer The Little Children
the battle against childhood cancer
by Dr. Jocelyn Joseph Demers

Translated by James Parry

ISBN: 0-920792-62-6

©1986 Eden Press

Cover design: Luba Zagurak
Page design: Evelyne Hertel

Printed in Canada at Metropole Litho Inc.
Dépôt légal — deuxième trimestre 1986
Bibliothèque nationale du Québec

Eden Press
4626 St. Catherine Street W.
Montreal, Québec H3Z 1S3
Canada

Canadian Cataloguing in Publication Data

Demers, Jocelyn
  Suffer the little children : the battle
against childhood cancer

Translation of: Victimes du cancer mais— des
enfants comme les autres.
ISBN 0-920792-62-6

1. Tumors in children. 2. Tumors in children—
Psychological aspects. 3. Tumors in children—
Biography. I. Title.

RJ416.L4D4513 1986   618.92'994   C86-090134-3

Grown-ups never understand anything on their own. And it is tiring for children always having to explain things to them.
— Antoine de Saint-Exupéry,
from The Little Prince

To my wife

A TRIBUTE

There are great numbers of researchers and clinical physicians who persist in trying to discover a cure for cancer. Some of these men and women are exceptionally gifted people. The majority, however, are people who are extraordinary only in that they have devoted their lives to medicine. In doing so, they have sacrificed their own comforts and sometimes even their health. They are indefatigable fighters who will drive themselves to the very limit in experimenting with a new treatment or on a research project. They work in the shadows and in anonymity. They work and will continue to work in search of a discovery that is perhaps small in appearance, but that will permit medical science to take a giant leap forward.

These fighters in the shadows deserve our admiration and our gratitude. I have been fortunate during my career to meet several of them, but Dr. Myron Karon will always have a very special place in my memory. This small, rotund man was recognized as one of the top practitioners in the field of cancer in children. He was loved, respected, and even held in awe throughout America and Europe. At the time I knew him he was director of the hematology-oncology department at the Los Angeles Children's Hospital, attached to the University of Southern California. Before being appointed to this post he had, like many other researchers, worked hard with patients and had completed several research projects. He had published numerous articles dealing with the effects of certain drugs, most notably analogues of purines and pyrimidines. All of these articles bore witness to the intensive research he had undertaken during eight years at the National Cancer Institute at Bethesda and at the M.D. Anderson Hospital and Tumor Institute in Houston.

Not only was Dr. Karon respected by all of his colleagues, he was also adored by his patients. To them, he was a sort of god. He gave them unshakeable confidence. This man led an extraordinarily full life. He could be found in Houston during the morning, Washington in the afternoon, and in his office in Los Angeles the following morning. Somehow, he still managed to find time to make sure his department was running smoothly, to keep a close eye on the research projects, and to become involved with clinical problems directly related to the care of cancerous children. Despite these incredible responsibilities, he knew the importance of giving the best of himself to his wife and three children. He discussed religion and philosophy with them. Whenever time allowed, he would take his family for a few hours of fishing in the Pacific. He also played the flute.

Dr. Karon was only 42 when a cerebral hemorrhage abruptly ended his life; a life that had been so full and happy. A week before this tragedy, I witnessed a scene that had a profound effect on me. Jackie, a 17-year-old black girl, was suffering from an osteosarcoma. Numerous metastases had attacked her lungs. She was aware of what had happened and she realized that her chances of recovery were virtually nil. Nothing short of a miracle could save her.

She had never stopped believing in Dr. Karon, but that day she was particularly depressed and was unable to hold back her tears. She looked into his eyes and said, "I'm going to die, aren't I?" The kindly doctor, who was known to be incapable of telling a lie, lowered his head. After a long silence, he put his hand on the young girl's shoulder and said simply, "So am I, some day." Jackie responded with a smile. She understood that she had to continue to fight, that truly, where there is life there is hope, that nothing is definite or forever. Jackie died a few weeks later, never knowing that her doctor departed from this world just ten days after their conversation.

During his short career, Dr. Karon passed on the sacred flame to other young doctors who now labour to realize his dream; to find a cure that will eliminate or at least check cancer. It is a cruel disease that strikes indiscriminately, even those we love most dearly, our children. These young researchers and doctors are following the example set by Dr. Karon.

They labour in our hospitals. You only have to look for them, although they almost always work away from the public eye. You could almost believe that they don't exist, but their work, their results, and their successes guarantee that they will never be forgotten. One cannot see the ripples in a pond unless someone has thrown in a stone. The ripples are the progress made in understanding cancer; they are the result of the stones thrown by these dedicated people who ask only for our help.

ACKNOWLEDGEMENTS

I first began writing this book almost six years ago and I often wondered whether it would ever see the light of day. During this time, I was able to count on the generous collaboration of several people, whom I would now like to thank.

I would like to express my gratitude to Stuart Siegel for the pleasure with which he undertook writing the preface for this volume.

Suzanne Douesnard, psychologist, was kind enough to write a chapter on the interior drama experienced by leukemic and cancerous children. She has supported me throughout this long project. My sincere thanks, Suzanne.

Doctors Arié Bensoussan, chief of surgery at Sainte-Justine Hospital, and Flore Fournelle-Lebuis, radiotherapist at Nôtre-Dame Hospital, have kindly collaborated on those pages touching on their respective specialties. My thanks to you both.

I would also like to pay tribute to the parents of Eric, to Michele, to all my young friends at the clinic, and to their parents for having given me permission to write so freely of their lives.

My thanks to the medical team, my colleagues, and to all those who create and animate the extraordinary world I have tried to reveal in these pages.

I would like to say a very special thank you to my wife, Gigi, for her unfailing help and support during all the time I worked on the book.

Finally I would like to thank my children, François, Elisabeth and Stéphanie. In bringing constant joy to my life, they have enabled me better to understand the drama that all parents of leukemic or cancerous children share, parents whom I come into contact with every day at Sainte-Justine Hospital.

J. Demers

TABLE OF CONTENTS

PREFACE

As Dr. Demers notes, the world of childhood cancer is full of people just like you and me. Yet only brief glimpses of this world have been made public, and these images have usually been through the eyes of anguished parents putting down on paper, often with simple eloquence, the individual experiences they have had during the illnesses of their children. Talented writers have given us more detached "human interest" stories.

In this book, Dr. Demers combines a clear yet detailed description of the technical aspects of childhood cancer and its treatment with a number of unique perspectives of the real drama, triumphs and tragedies experienced every day. Particularly special are the recollections of Michele, a young woman looking back on her fight against leukemia. What she and the other children we are privileged to meet tell us about how much they understand about serious illness, and how important honesty is in relating to children, should not be forgotten by physicians, nurses, and parents alike.

Perhaps the most important contribution that Dr. Demers makes in this book, however, is the view of this "battlefield" and the courage of the combatants that we gain through the eyes of the physician and medical research team who provide the major "ammunition" in this fight. Dr. Demers is certainly in a perfect position to provide us with these insights. First choosing a career in medicine and then in pediatrics, he made the difficult decision to train in the pediatric specialty that cares for the number-one killer of children aside from accidents—cancer.

Why do people choose to deal with dying children, angry and despondent parents, and frustrating medical problems that fail to respond like the medical textbooks and their training say they should? Dr. Demers shows us why on almost every page of this book. How many people have the opportunity, and the privilege, to observe "real-life" human courage every day of their lives? And how many of us have the opportunity to play a personal role in triumphing over deadly illnesses and in trying to advance the frontiers of our knowledge about these killers to gain even more important keys to the secrets that will provide the ultimate victory? Dr. Demers has given the reader the chance to share in both the pain and frustration as well as the exhilaration that members of the medical-care team experience every day. Through his eyes, patients, families and the general public will gain a greater understanding of how the battle against childhood cancer is really being fought.

Stuart Elliott Siegel, M.D.
Head, Division of Hematology-Oncology
Children's Hospital of Los Angeles
Los Angeles, California

FOREWORD

A child looks at you
with eyes full of wonder.
And a smile is born.

His tiny arms reach out.
And in a twinkling of an eye,
he jumps
to be cradled in yours,
full of confidence
and crying out for love.

There is nothing that can be done.
You are trapped.
Worries, misfortune, sickness,
are forgotten.
And without knowing why,
you smile.
To become more childlike than the
child.

When I wrote this naive poem I was 16 years old. It was my first, and almost my last, attempt at poetry. I didn't know then that the subject I had chosen so instinctively would come to determine my entire future. At that moment I didn't know that my life would be linked in a very special way with children. I could not predict that after having worked as a doctor at a hospital for sick children in Africa, I would become a pediatrician-hematologist in my own country. Or that, in this way, I would come to devote the greater part of my life to taking care of children suffering from cancer.

It is no secret that life is full of surprises. I am convinced that if you remain faithful to your youthful ambitions, and if luck is on your side, those dreams can become a reality. At an early age I dreamed of helping others, of giving the best of myself to them.

My experiences in Africa, from 1967 to 1970, had a profound effect on me. Fresh from the so-called civilized world of the privileged, which so many of us take for granted, I was suddenly confronted with human misery and suffering of unbelievable magnitude. It was a devastating and extremely painful introduction to an unknown world. I was surrounded by victims of total deprivation while I, for my part, was able to continue a normal life. I did not have to live with the gnawing pangs of hunger eating away at me every day. I did not have to try and sleep through the chillingly cold, damp nights of winter in an unheated home. This poverty remains with us today; more than twelve million children throughout the world die of hunger every year. Many agencies have compiled statistics on the causes of death among children. They speak knowledgeably of pneumonia, measles, poliomyelitis, malaria, gastroentritis, and so on, but all of these causes are merely accelerating factors. In reality, the majority of these children are basically undernourished. They are rachitic, lacking in proteins, vitamins and iron. They are easy prey for sickness and disease.

When on duty in the emergency department or elsewhere in the hospital, I would use my stethoscope on hundreds of children in just a few short hours. Each one was as ill as the next, but my role was limited to admitting only those suffering to a degree that threatened to be imminently fatal. I had to choose among the most severe cases. The others were sent home. We could merely advise them to report to their local clinic the next day. We knew only too well that the same scene would be repeated there, and that an in-depth study of their cases would be postponed until a later date.

The hospital had three hundred beds and they were always full. We were handicapped from the very start; we just did not have the space. To make matters worse, we had only a limited supply of drugs, some antibiotics, aspirin, and intravenous solutions for those who were dehydrated. At certain times of the year we lacked even these few palliatives. We had to resign ourselves to treating only the "most curable." The others, for whom treatment was postponed, were often beyond saving. What helplessness we all experienced!

One of my first nights on duty—I will never forget it—I lost nine children. I cried, discouraged. I hurt, feeling despair that I had never experienced before. I could not understand what was happening. My North American training had taught me to do everything humanly possible to save lives. This one night taught me that devotion and the will to succeed were not enough. It took personnel and materials to care for sick children, particularly those in an acute condition. How could we ever hope to win without first attacking the source, the cause of all this misery—malnutrition and lack of hygiene. The cure for this was beyond our control. All we could do was close our eyes, shut our ears, and bite our tongues. My university studies had not prepared me for this.

Of the young patients admitted to the hospital, some 20 percent died. When a child died, the only people at the bedside to witness the death were the nurse and the doctor. The parents were not permitted to enter the hospital. They were only allowed to see their child at a predetermined hour through a window looking out onto the courtyard. Deep suffering was caused by this lack of compassion. It was then and only then that the parents would be told of their child's death. What tears, what weeping and wailing and gnashing of teeth. The parents' only right was to carry away the tiny, lifeless body. The mothers were beside themselves with grief. Some of them sat on the ground wailing as they tried to squeeze now useless milk from their breasts. Others beat their breasts or scratched their faces with their nails to show their despair. In so-called civilized societies we have lost the ability to express our emotions so openly. Reason is made to prevail over emotion. Such tragic scenes, however, have much to teach us about ourselves and others, for they remind us of the very roots of our human nature.

These three years in Africa were, for me, a revelation. They represented my initiation to the world of human suffering. The strong revulsion and anger they created within me prepared me for a life of caring for other children—children in our own world who suffer from cancer. All of these children, those living in misery and hopelessness in Africa, and those living in relative comfort and prosperity in North America, proved one thing to me. Their courage and determination in the face of such cruel adversity is identical, despite the thousands of kilometers that separate them. Heroism is the same everywhere. It has only one face.

Cancer among children is a difficult reality to accept and live with. In the following chapters you will share with me moments of pain and even despair, but you will also experience moments of exultation. These pages tell the stories of children who fight a continuing battle against an invisible enemy, an enemy that embraces their very beings. Whether they are victorious or whether they are vanquished, they all share the same courage in their fight.

In this book I wish to pay tribute to the valour of the young people under my care; to their inestimable resources of patience, hope, and confidence—which they never lose; and also to their moral and physical courage. Truly, they deserve to be called heroes. I hope I have found the words to do justice to their battle and also to awaken love and compassion for these children in you. They are children who have been forced by blind fate to face death before they have ever lived. These young heroes are not fictional. They live among us and they sing—each in his or her own way—with all their strength, of the joy of life.

one

ERIC'S STORY

Joliette, Quebec, 10 November 1976. A child is born. His parents bend over the crib trying to predict his future, his destiny. Will he become one of those great thinkers capable of changing the course of history? Will be become one of those who create poetry, devoting himself to the magic of words? Or a composer of symphonies to stir the soul? The father and mother watch over their first-born with love and compassion. Yes, they tell themselves, this child, so confident and peaceful, and so innocent, this child they adore, will be a winner in every sense of the word.

Eric grew up. He was handsome and gracious. Watching him grow with such ease and good fortune, one would have believed the world was created just for him. He succeeded in everything he did. Always happy and in a good mood, he was like a little god whom nobody could refuse.

At the age of four he developed an exceptional interest in the stars. For him, the sun and moon belonged to the same world as the toy robot given him by his grandfather. Grampa was his favourite companion. He was someone who knew all the secrets of nature because every day he worked with plants at the Botanical Gardens. He was a man blessed with infinite patience. He and Eric were inseparable; two friends sharing all their joys and discoveries.

When Eric was eight fate dealt a cruel blow to the special relationship that had illuminated his childhood. Grampa died suddenly, following a brief illness. Eric took it very hard, feeling abandoned by a friend to whom he had given all his faith and love. However, he quickly came to an understanding of death and, through his tears, told his mother, "Mom, I know now. Grampa has gone to a better world. And I'll go there too some day."

The months, the seasons passed. Eric never forgot his grandfather, but his father, mother, younger sister and friends filled his universe. He joined a Wolf Cub Pack. He loved to join in team games and activities. He began to play hockey; he loved the game.

During a match in February, 1978, a scrimmage broke out in the goal area. The youngsters piled pell-mell onto the ice. Eric, who fell on top of his own goalie, got up complaining of pains in his legs and chest. He left the rink and headed home. A couple of hours later, his parents took him to the hospital for a check-up. There were no broken bones, but the doctor detected a high fever that he couldn't explain. He decided to keep Eric under observation. It appeared the simple accident was not, in itself, the cause of Eric's discomfort. He was kept in for seven days, during which time the doctors concluded the fever was caused, in all probability, by a viral infection or a lung inflammation. There was even the possibility of the beginning of rheumatoid arthritis. There were signs of improvement, however, and Eric was discharged.

He was never to feel well again. For more than two months he suffered from various complaints, ranging from tiredness to pains in various parts of his body. He lost weight. His mother and father became extremely worried and didn't know what to make of the laboratory tests that failed to reveal anything serious.

By the beginning of May, Eric had grown increasingly pale. His mother decided to consult the doctor again. The doctor, convinced that the case was becoming more disturbing, decided to re-admit the child.

"Doctor," said the mother, "nothing is going like it was before. What's wrong with him? What has he got?"

"I don't know. Your son still has a fever, but his blood count is very good."

"Doctor, I'm afraid. I'm afraid Eric has leukemia."

To reassure her, that very same day the doctor consulted with a blood-disease specialist. Perhaps this hematologist would shed some light on the mystery. Uncertainties raced through the mother's mind while she waited for the results. Would he confirm her worst fears? She almost regretted having mentioned the word. She was afraid. The hematologist went ahead with his examination, which including tapping the bone marrow. Minutes turned into hours before the mother was to learn the results of these tests at a meeting with the specialist.

"Your son is suffering from leukemia. Our examinations leave no room for doubt. In Eric's case, it is an acute form of leukemia that is among the most difficult to treat. It is, therefore, one of the most serious."

The mother could hardly believe her ears. Had she heard right? Was the doctor serious? She didn't seem to react at all. No tears. No sobs. Only a sigh. She pinched herself to make sure she wasn't dreaming. Her child suffering from leukemia? It didn't seem possible.

Eric would have to be transferred to Sainte-Justine Hospital the following day. Sadly, the doctor explained what hospitalization involved, knowing full well how cruel his words must sound. Eric wasn't told the nature of his illness right away. His mother bore the terrible weight alone. His father would soon be finishing work and would arrive at the hospital for the visiting hours. What would she tell her husband when he arrived, tired and worn out after a hard day's work? How would he take the news? She decided not to tell him anything when he arrived. She would wait until the visit was over so that he could spend a little more time with his son, in peace. When the time came she told him the truth. After a long heavy silence, the couple threw their arms around one another and wept uncontrollably.

The following morning, Eric was isolated from the other children. He couldn't understand what was happening. He cried. Meanwhile, the doctor began arranging for the transfer. At about one in the afternoon, he told the parents they must leave immediately, with Eric, for Montreal. The staff at Sainte-Justine was waiting for them. It was about two when Eric got in the car. He didn't want to leave for Montreal before stopping at school to say hello to the friends he hadn't seen for ten days. They were all playing in the schoolyard. Eric talked to them for a while and then suggested to his parents that they stop by the house. He wanted to see the apple trees in bloom at the bottom of the garden, and to have a quick look around his room to make sure everything was as he had left it. This done, he turned to his mother and said, "Mommy, rock me in your arms, will you?"

His mother was shaken. It had been a long time since Eric had curled up in her lap. Yet today he wanted to rediscover the warmth of his mother's arms. She held him tightly. "Daddy, pour me a glass of soda pop." Contented, his small wishes fulfilled, they set out for Montreal. In doing so, Eric and his parents were taking the first steps on a long and difficult road through an unknown and threatening world.

A young intern was waiting for them when they arrived at their destination five hours later.

"We were expecting you earlier. We were told at noon that you'd be arriving soon."

"We had a few things to do before . . ." stammered the mother, not wanting to admit that she and her husband had wanted Eric to have a few moments of freedom before bringing him to the hospital.

"That's fine. Doctor R. will be along to see you a little later. While we're waiting, why don't you tell me how it all started."

And so it began. There was no escaping the fact that Eric had a serious illness. He had to receive treatment, and he had to be cured. Yes, they were reassured, Eric would win his fight against cancer. He had to. The hematologist on duty arrived a little later. He had already done a microscopic study of the bone marrow smear that had been delivered to him earlier. He now examined his patient very carefully.

"Eric, we're going to take very good care of you," he said on finishing his examination. "But right now I need to talk to your parents. It will be the only time we don't talk in front of you. I'll come back right away."

Eric agreed, and a few minutes later, the parents met with Dr. R. in his office.

"You know what's happening, don't you."
"Yes. Eric is suffering from an acute form of leukemia," replied the father.
"That's right. We have to agree with the diagnosis made by the doctors in Joliette. We've examined the bone marrow sample. Your son has an acute myeloblastic leukemia. It's a form that's very difficult to treat."

The discussion then turned to the nature of the illness, its probable causes, complications, possible treatments, their advantages, and the possible unpleasant side effects. The doctor promised to come back to each of the subjects and discuss them in greater detail in the days that followed.

"Doctor, will he suffer?" asked the mother.
"Yes, but we intend to do everything possible to minimize the pain."
"Have you already cured children suffering from this kind of leukemia?"
"Yes, I remember two cases—"
"Good. Then Eric will be the third, doctor. He will get better."

Only after this discussion was Eric told the true nature of his illness, as well as about the treatment he was going to receive, beginning immediately. The word *leukemia* did not seem to disturb him too much. All the same, he asked a question that startled both the doctor and his parents.

"Can I die from this illness?"

"Eric, you're very ill, but we'll do all we can to make you better."

"Then I will get better," declared the youngster with a big smile.

And so the treatment began on an optimistic note. Eric knew that he would be feeling very poorly, that he would probably lose his hair. He also realized how important the stakes were, and declared that nothing was going to stop him from getting better.

The first weeks of treatment passed quickly. Eric was increasingly encouraged. His parents could not forget, however, that their son was seriously ill, though they never let their emotions show in front of him. In the eyes of their own parents and friends, and of the doctors and hospital staff, they were towers of strength. They were brave and courageous people. It was Eric, however, who set the example. It was Eric, in fact, who supported them.

Treatment progressed to the fourth stage. More than six weeks had passed since the diagnosis. Eric was holding up well and, to the surprise of the new hematologist on duty, the blood count was well within normal limits. He decided to make another test of the bone marrow to discover what was happening there. Eric prepared himself with a certain apprehension. But he already felt so much better that he was convinced the bone marrow would also be back to normal. "Eric, I have great news for you," said the doctor on entering the boy's room.

Eric's mother hung on the doctor's every word. Eric looked at his mother, his eyes shining, waiting for the one word that would allow him to leave the hospital and regain his freedom:

"Eric, you have a remission."

"Hurray! Let's go home!"

"Not so fast, in a little while."

The atmosphere in the room had changed completely with this first victory. It was, hopefully, the first step towards a final victory. Eric was overjoyed and his mother was all smiles. They began to bargain with the doctor.

"Perhaps we could—"

"Eric, today you'll get only one injection. We'll give you all the medicine in one shot. As soon as we've finished, you can go home. However, you must continue your treatment at home. Take your medicine every day."

"I will, I will, I promise."

He jumped out of bed, looked out the window, and thought of Joliette. A few hours later he was there. The only thing he wanted to do was to meet his father at work. He wanted to tell him the fantastic news right away. "Eric! What are you doing here?" The boy jumped into his father's arms and gave him a big hug. "Guess what, Daddy. I have a remission!" It was just like Christmas, and what a Christmas at that. It was a thousand times more beautiful than all the other Christmases put together.

Eric returned regularly to the outpatient clinic of the hematology department; eventually these visits became less and less frequent. He revelled in his new-found freedom and his gradually returning strength. As he had begun to lose his hair, little by little, he took to wearing a cap—as much to hide his baldness as to avoid embarrassing questions. The moment arrived when he had to submit to treatment designed primarily as a preventive measure: radiation of the brain. The purpose of this treament is to destroy any leukemic cells that have lodged in the brain or in the fluid surrounding it, and also to avoid a relapse in this area. This radiotherapy is accompanied by four to six spinal taps at weekly intervals. These taps are the most painful part of the treatment. They serve to take samples of the spinal fluid for study and also to inject a powerful anti-leukemic drug that, when combined with X-rays, can enhance the ability to kill any leukemic cells hiding out in this sanctuary. Eric's parents feared this part of the treatment. They knew they had to drive him to Nôtre-Dame Hospital in Montreal, five times a week for two to three weeks. What worried them more than anything else was how their son would face up to this new test and to the total baldness that followed it.

Eric was impressed by the huge radiation machines, and during his first sessions he felt a little threatened by them. The minutes he spent with them seemed like hours, but he quickly overcame his fears. As they bombarded him with X-rays, he came to accept them as companions of the road. He soon had his old confidence back.

In the weeks that followed, our young friend lost all his hair. It didn't seem to upset him too much because he knew that the baldness was only temporary. His mother tried to encourage him, as only a mother can. "Eric, you have beautiful eyes. And such a big heart!"

Eric laughed. All the same, he was never seen without his little cap. The only things that embarrassed him were indiscreet or awkward questions from adults. In August, he was asked at the last minute to be an altar boy at the wedding of one of his aunts. The officiating priest, who had not been informed of Eric's illness, saw him arriving, all smiles, but wearing a cap in church.

"You are in the house of God. Won't you take off your hat?"
"It's part of my normal dress," Eric replied, not put out in the least.

The priest did not press the issue. The boy's firm reply and the look of vexation on his face made the priest realize that Eric had his own good reasons for wearing the cap. That same day, one of the wedding guests also remarked on the cap. This time, Eric's mother was there to help him out. She simply looked at the woman without saying a word. Then, very calmly, she lifted her son's cap just enough to reveal the absence of hair on his head. The silence that followed spoke volumes. The guest stammered an apology, and after an awkward silence, conversations resumed. Eric went off to play with children his own age. For them, his baldness was not a problem. It only took a few words to strike up a relationship that in more than one instance, was the beginning of a lasting friendship.

Several weeks passed. Eric was once again full of life. He was glowing with health and could hardly wait to return to school. His parents looked on this return as a new test. How would Eric, who had become the life and soul of the party, be greeted by his former classmates? Would they look on him as a clown because of his baldness. As a sad object of curiosity? Would he be made to suffer because of their unwitting cruelty? As it turned out, these fears were unfounded. Eric returned to the fifth grade. So he had fallen behind his age group a little, what did it matter? The important thing was that he could join the same group of friends after class for play.

The days passed quickly. One day in November, as luck would have it the word *cancer* cropped up during class. The teacher, a little embarrassed, asked the pupils what they knew and what they thought about the illness. Only a few ventured to say anything. They spoke vaguely of an aunt or an uncle who had died of an illness something like cancer. In reality, they didn't know a lot about it and seemed uncomfortable discussing it. Then Eric stood up and described the illness that had affected him. He described it as an acute myeloblastic leukemia, a cancer of the blood. Every once in a while he would throw in other technical medical terms. He spoke at fair length of the treatment he was undergoing. His bald head was proof for everyone to see. He finished by saying, "I'll get over this illness. I want to become a researcher and work to find the cause of leukemia. I want to treat other kids who are suffering from leukemia like me."

Eric earned some precious points that day. He also won an out-pouring of sympathy and admiration. Even more importantly, perhaps, he gained the support of the boys and girls in his school. Now everyone wanted to get behind him in his battle; they wanted to share in his dream of becoming a researcher.

The months passed and winter drew to a close. In mid-March, after yet another examination at the outpatient's clinic, Dr. R. took Eric's mother by the arm and invited her to follow him to a nearby office.

"Eric is doing so well, doctor. What's the matter?"

"His blood count is no longer normal. It's very painful for me to say this, but Eric is having a relapse."

"That can't be. Do some more tests. It's impossible, impossible!"

"He might look healthy, but the facts don't lie. He's suffering from a relapse. And he has a right to know what's happening."

What did all this mean to Eric? A relapse? Perhaps more chemotherapy? Even more serious for Eric was the possibility of not being able to attend winter camp with the Cubs the following week. There was no way that Eric wanted to miss that, and so he began negotiating: "You can do anything you want to me as long as you let me go to camp."

A bargain was struck. Eric received a transfusion and a new form of chemotherapy called Cytosar. Delivered in high doses, it inevitably causes nausea and vomiting.

"Am I going to lose my hair again?"

"Perhaps a little, Eric, but not completely."

"Oof," sighed Eric, obviously relieved.

Would March 13 mark the beginning of a new black period in Eric's life? Would he become ill all over again because of the new drugs? Would it be necessary to give him transfusions to keep his blood count at an acceptable level? The questions could not yet be answered. What was known was that before going to camp, he would have to attend the outpatient clinic for five days. Wasn't that painful enough? Such were the questions Eric's mother asked herself on this black day. What would her husband say when he heard the news? She made a promise to herself. Whatever else happened, Eric would go to camp. There he would have a short time in which to forget the chemotherapy he would soon have to face. He was going to enjoy himself.

From the beginning of April, Eric attended the outpatient clinic. Blood tests revealed that, while fewer in number, the leukemic cells were still present. A change was taking place in our young friend, who had been so brave up to this point. The simple routine of injections became a difficult and laborious operation. They became painful. Sometimes Eric took several minutes to convince himself that he shouldn't pull his arm away when the needle approached. The medical team talked to him, trying to encourage him, trying to give him all the moral support he needed. They even brought in a psychologist in the hope that discussing the problem would help Eric to allay his fears. Unfortunately, even this didn't work: "I know the needle won't hurt me, but I can't help it. I'm afraid."

Everyone was concerned and alarmed. This young man, who had always been so brave, was now hopelessly afraid when it came time for an injection. He often pulled his arm away, crying out in fear. It took an hour, sometimes two, to administer a single injection. The medical staff was at a loss as to what to do. Medication to reduce anxiety, psychotherapy, even hypnosis, were all useless. Nothing worked. The only solution that remained was to forcibly restrain Eric. Two or three people held his arms so that he couldn't pull away. After it was over, he'd calm down almost immediately. He would smile and be his normal self again, while the doctors, nurses and parents were drained by the ordeal. They felt guilty and miserable. Eric, once again in a cheerful mood, would console them. He'd tell them what he had planned for tomorrow or the next week. For him the crisis was over. He was only afraid. For the adults, there was already concern for the next time. Would this start all over again when it came time for the next injection?

Apart from these crises, Eric took everything in stride. May arrived, and Eric was to be Confirmed this month. In addition, his parents told him of a marvellous adventure they had planned for him: a trip to Disneyworld in Florida. Eric could think of nothing else but these two events. His parents were suddenly worried. Had they promised him something that was simply out of the question at the moment? Should they wait for another remission?

"What do you think, doctor?" the father asked.
"It's an excellent idea. We must do everything we can to ensure that he's in good shape for this holiday. You shouldn't wait too long, however, because it's possible Eric will have to confront some major problems three or four weeks from now. We'll orient our treatment in such a way as to let him enjoy a holiday in the enchanted kingdom."

The parents now realized that time had become an important factor. They asked themselves what the doctor's words really meant. Surely he was exaggerating. They felt sure Eric was going to have a remission any day now.

The Confirmation took place one beautiful evening in May. Eric was well prepared. He knew that this sacrament was going to make him a soldier of Christ. He'd recently seen a television program on the life of Martin Luther King. For Eric, the civil rights leader had become a symbol of courage. He was Eric's hero, and Eric wanted to be like him. "I also want to be a true Christian. And, after my death, I will go to be closer to God," he told his parents one evening.

His parents were alarmed. Why was he talking about dying? They knew that Eric had changed since the relapse. He had become more thoughtful. He seemed to spend a lot of time daydreaming. He seemed distant. On several occasions he told them that he was afraid of dying. This last confidence betrayed the deep anxiety he was feeling.

Two days after his Confirmation, he was to leave for Florida. The big day had arrived, the dream had become reality. His parents stocked up with all the necessary drugs, just in case the worst should happen. As for Eric, he was more concerned about what time they would land in Orlando. It was going to be so good to get far, far away from the hospital and all those doctors. He was determined not to miss a thing at Disneyworld. The birds of paradise, the pirates of yesteryear, and the astronauts of the future filled his imagination and populated his fantasy world. Yet, of all the things that he saw during that trip, it was the sea that fascinated him the most. It was love at first sight. He threw himself into the water as if discovering a long-lost friend. After swimming, he dried himself off and sat for a long time, deep in thought as the waves broke gently on the sand. Clearly, he was experiencing something profound; he was like someone possessed.

"Eric, that's enough. You mustn't take too much sun on the first day. It can make you sick."
"Don't worry, Mommy, nothing's going to happen."

And nothing did. Eric was up at the crack of dawn the next day. He dressed and hurried out to meet his new friend, the sea.

The week flew by. All good things must come to an end and it was time to go home. The dream had ended, soon to be replaced by harsh reality. As soon as he returned, he would have to begin treatment all over again. Those damn needles would once again pierce his skin, skin that was now tanned and revitalized. Eric resigned himself to the inevitable, but not without making a few faces. Not without repeating that he was afraid. Not without frequently saying that it was all too much for him.

Then Eric had a remission—at least it appeared so because the leukemic cells had disappeared from his blood stream. He finished the school year in great form. Despite the many days he had missed, he passed the fifth grade in remarkable fashion. His teachers had nothing but praise for his work and his behaviour in general. In July, Eric left for camp again. While there he loved to play the role of Caesar, deciding which of his subjects would live and which would die. But Caesar seemed paler and more tired than usual.

After camp, Eric returned to the hospital, where he was in for a nasty surprise. He had had a second relapse. The remission, probably only a partial one, had not lasted. It was a terrible blow. What was he going to do now? What was the point in going on? How was he going to find the strength to fight all over again? The hematologists conferred and decided to go for broke, to play their trump card. As Eric was not responding to chemotherapy, they would resort to a new method of treatment that was still in an experimental stage. They would use a brand new drug that was strongly recommended after testing in the laboratory, but which had only been in use on humans for a few months at this point. After a long discussion with the parents, a hematologist spoke to Eric.

"Eric, are you willing to try a new medicine, 5-AZA-2'-deoxycytidine?"

"Five what?" asked Eric.

"Five-AZA."

"Is it going to make me lose my hair? Is it going to make me sick? I hope I can swallow it and not have to have a needle."

"Sorry, Eric, but we'll have to use a needle. It's got to be injected, but none of the children who've taken it so far have had any bad side effects."

Eric was once again encouraged. He could dream again. A drug still in the experimental stage would give him the chance to meet the researchers. He still wanted to join their team one day.

Everything was prepared in the next few hours. A blood sample was taken, as well as a sample of the bone marrow to determine whether the leukemic cells were susceptible to the new treatment. The results were positive. Eric received an intravenous injection of 5-AZA. It took an hour. Our young friend left the hospital feeling calm and confident.

He had to return in eight days as the treatment had to be repeated every week until there was a detectable improvement.

By August 17, after four weeks of treatment, the dosage was doubled. The leukemic cells had not responded the doctors had hoped and so they decided to give him another dose, but over a longer period of time. The perfusion lasted eight hours instead of one. When Eric returned to the hospital ten days later, he had a stubborn cough. An X-ray of his lungs indicated pneumonia; he would have to be hospitalized.

"Eric, you're going to stay with us for a while. You're going to be given antibiotics. I'm sorry, but they have to be by needle."

"Oh no, not again! My veins can't take any more."

There was no choice, and so Eric was admitted. In the days that followed, pneumonia took over his poor, wracked body. The antibiotics no longer seemed to have any effect, probably because there were no white blood cells and the leukemic cells were raging unchecked. His condition worsened daily, but Eric fought back, always asking when he could leave the hospital. It was impossible. The doctors and consultants treating Eric decided to proceed with a lung biopsy in order to determine the exact nature of the pneumonia. Could it be a bacterial infection? Fungus? Or an invasion of the lung tissue by malignant cells? Eric agreed to the biopsy, even though he knew that he really had no choice in the matter. He admitted that he was afraid, and everyone did their best to reassure him. The biopsy performed on September 5 verified the infectious nature of the pneumonia. The antibiotics were changed accordingly, but the question of whether something more sinister was lurking in the background remained. Could it be that the leukemia was slyly taking on an unusual form?

In the weeks that followed, Eric became more and more dyspneic. He seemed to be suffocating. The doctors feared the worst, and Eric was transferred to intensive care. His parents paced the floor for hours. What were all those doctors doing in his room? Could they really do anything? Could Eric keep up his courage? The long, painful hours dragged by. Eric was suffering and could no longer make himself understood. He was on artifical respiration now, his hands and feet connected to tubes that fed him and supplied him with painkillers.

"The illness is stronger than he is. Eric isn't improving," the doctor told his parents.

"No, you'll see," replied Eric's mother. Emphatically she added, "You don't really know Eric. He's a winner, he'll get better."

Eric drifted in and out of consciousness, his breathing difficult and irregular. He required strong sedatives. Even in this state, one could feel him flinching, trying to escape, when anyone approached him with a needle. What could be done to make him understand that everyone was with him? Only his mother's hand on his arm could calm him. The doctor explained the situation to Eric's parents, who were now starting to feel powerless.

"Nothing is going as we would like it to, but we're doing everything we possibly can. There's no doubt that the pneumonia has a leukemic component. The level of leukemic cells in his blood is now more than sixty percent. We'd like to try again with a stronger dose of 5-AZA, but this time we'll administer it over a thirty-six hour period. The drug will act directly on the leukemia and indirectly, we hope, on the pneumonia. There is a risk of side effects, but we won't know for sure for another two to four weeks. What we have to do now is get Eric out of this stalemate. What do you think?"

"Do everything you can for him, doctor. We have faith in you."

The conversation, which had seemed so removed from reality, ended there. The 5-AZA was prepared, the special pump set in place, and the drug administered. Everyone was hoping for a miracle. The very next day saw signs of improvement, which became even more pronounced in the days that followed. Eric had pulled through yet again. Everyone was full of hope. His parents never lost faith; they knew their son. Eric made such incredible progress that he left intensive care for his own room. All was quiet and peaceful. His lungs had cleared up. The number of leukemic cells had dropped considerably, and Eric became more and more optimistic. It was inevitable, however, that such a traumatic experience would leave scars. Eric had difficulty in speaking and his coordination was off. He also walked with difficulty, but in the weeks that followed he made a miraculous recovery.

On September 20, his mother's birthday, Eric was chatting with her and Suzanne, the psychologist who had been helping him since he first became ill. He told them of a strange dream he had had during the days he battled against pneumonia:

"I was in heaven, and I saw Grampa, who took me by the hand and told me that I was going to beat my pneumonia. He was covered by a shadow and I couldn't really see his face. The Lord stood before me and told me that I was going back to earth. It was beautiful in heaven. Everything was so bright. There was light everywhere, but I couldn't see where it was coming from. I was so relaxed, I was floating. I wasn't tied down by tubes. I was free, and I didn't want to come back. You know, I'm not afraid of dying anymore. I know that everything is good up there and that everyone's happy in heaven."

Eric's mother was deeply moved. He had described his dream so clearly and now exuded such inner peace and calm that his mother and the psychologist wondered whether he had in fact come back from some other world. They had never seen him so self-assured. From that day on, Eric retained this beautiful serenity.

Eric was firmly convinced that he would beat his illness. He again declared he would become a researcher, devoting his life to fighting those illnesses that the doctors were now unable to cure.

Another Christmas approached. During the last two months, Eric's condition had remained relatively stable. He was living at home, but returned twice a week to the hospital to have his blood count checked. Since the bout with pneumonia he had received two doses of 5-AZA, both over a period of forty hours. The number of leukemic cells varied, but it seemed impossible at this time to eliminate them altogether. The healthy platelets and the hemoglobin levels dropped regularly. They dropped so much and so often that transfusions were now a frequent necessity.

Finally Christmas arrived. "Mommy, Daddy, we've spent some beautiful Christmases together, but this is the best one ever." This Christmas was different from all those that had gone before. Eric was at peace. He listened to a record that he had come to love: "Jonathan Livingston Seagull." Even though the words were in English, Eric, who only spoke French, seemed to understand everything. Wasn't this seagull who wanted to achieve the impossible a symbol of the heroic battle that our young friend was fighting against a relentless enemy?

On January 3, 1980, Eric's parents were once again called in to the hematologist's office. Their son was suffering from severe pains in his bones, just as he had at the beginning of his illness. His blood count was far from good, he was suffering from severe anemia, and he was hemorrhaging. It was hoped that blood and platelet transfusions would remedy the problem. The hematologist wondered whether it would be better to return to chemotherapy in its conventional form or to continue with the 5-AZA in the hope that this time it would give better results. Eric's parents were at a loss as to what to answer when this question was put to them. What experience did they have to equip them to decide between the two options? What other choice did they have but to accept the recommendation of the doctors and agree to the one that the professionals felt offered the best chance of success? Their real fear was that the day would come when the doctors would have nothing to propose because nothing more could be done. This eventuality was something they just didn't want to think about.

Eric received another perfusion of 5-AZA. His condition improved greatly over the next few days and the pain disappeared. Even so, he had to submit to blood and platelet transfusions. He did not take to them well; his veins were in very bad shape. First it had been his lungs that refused to fight. Now his veins, those tiny blood vessels that are hardly visible and whose only function is to carry blood, rebelled in turn. They burst at the slightest touch and became irritated by any foreign substance injected into them.

On January 15, Eric was at home. It was a beautiful winter's day and he was in excellent spirits. During the day, he confided to his parents that he was not afraid of dying. That night, however, things took a turn for the worse. He cried and vomited. He bled slightly from the nose. Eric's parents were distraught. Despite the late hour, they decided to bring him to the hospital. He was getting worse by the minute. Was he merely sleeping or was he unconscious? The car was in the drive, but they thought it wiser to call an ambulance.

"Quick! Sainte-Justine Hospital in Montreal," the mother told the ambulance driver.

"But that's too far!"

"He'll make it."

The eighty kilometers to the hospital seemed like a thousand, despite the speed at which they were travelling. His mother clutched Eric's hand, though he was now unconscious. His father followed in the family car, heedless of the speed limit, the dangerous bends in the road, and the poor visibility. He knew that his son was in danger, more so than ever before.

Finally, they saw the lights of the hospital. The doctor on duty was by their side in seconds. It was a woman who knew Eric very well. She took one look at Eric and said, "He's probably lost some blood in the brain. Quick, we must give him a platelet transfusion!"

The hematologist on duty arrived immediately and confirmed the preliminary diagnosis.

"It looks like an intracranial hemorrhage. I'm afraid your son will be permanently affected by it."

"It's not true!" cried the boy's mother.

Eric's father left suddenly. In the corridor of the emergency room he began to sob, all the while striking the walls with all his strength. Usually so calm and collected, he could no longer hide the monstrous anguish that tortured him. He beat against the solid walls. Those around him tried to comfort him, to restrain him, but to no avail. Finally his wife rushed up and threw her arms around him. "That's enough!" He calmed down immediately. Even now, when everything seemed lost, they knew they had no right to give up, to lose control of themselves. It was time to pray. The priest arrived to give Eric the Last Rites.

They had to face reality. Eric was dying. Deep in her heart his mother remained hopeful. Eric was in a deep coma all the next day. He then seemed to recover a little. The neurologist detected an improvement in his reflexes; he could only marvel at the tenacity of this boy. To be still alive and fighting after such a serious cerebro-vascular attack was in itself extraordinary. A few hours later, Eric regained consciousness. The few words he spoke comforted and encouraged those around him.

"I want to see Mommy and Daddy." His mother was beside herself with joy. Eric had triumphed again. "Eric." "I have a headache and my neck hurts." The next two days proved conclusively that Eric was indeed suffering from intracranial hemorrhaging, which resulted in serious damage to his brain. Some slight improvement was still possible, but the hemorrhaging had taken its toll: Eric was blind. Fortunately, he was not really aware of what was happening to him. He was like a little child, crying out for tenderness.

"I'm in a big black hole. Mommy, Daddy, I love you. Where is my teddy bear?"

"Don't wear yourself out, Eric," whispered his mother. "You have to rest, your brain is ill. You're going through a rough time, but you must get through it."

Three days had passed since the vascular-cerebral attack. Despite some signs of clinical improvement, other problems had arisen. There was an intense rash—an allergic reaction to the morphine—that prompted Eric to scratch himself incessantly. His hands had to be wrapped in thick bandages to prevent him from hurting himself. The doctors suggested that he scratch the teddy bear when the itching became too unbearable, and he did.

One evening he had such a terrible headache that the morphine didn't help at all. Was he losing blood again? He was given a new perfusion of platelets. For the next two or three days, things were relatively calm. Eric still couldn't see, but at least he could talk to his parents. He asked whether they were taking care of Coco, his parrot. He asked about his friends and those he loved, Marie-Claude, Louise, Dick, Hortense, Marie, Suzanne, Emilien, and the others. He told them he didn't want to die. He wanted to become a famous doctor and not do harm to anyone. He even talked about going on his honeymoon. "But with who, Eric? And where?" "With you, mommy. To Hawaii."

Then things took a turn for the worse. Eric was suffering. His allergic reaction to the morphine continued. His body went into convulsions. He slipped in and out of consciousness as the hours dragged by. His body and spirit were locked in a final battle. He whispered:

"Mommy, have faith, because I do. I am sitting at my desk. I am a doctor. I'm doing research. I'm helping children to get better."

A few hours after speaking these words he passed on. Eric would suffer no more. It was January 25, 1980.

● ● ●

From the time of his first diagnosis, Eric's illness had lasted 628 days. He had spent one quarter of these days either in a hospital bed or visiting the doctors. He had received more than eight hundred blood tests, numerous spinal and bone-marrow taps, 30 X-rays, 120 biochemical tests, and more than two hundred transfusions. No fewer than twenty doctors—hematologists, pulmonologists, neurologists, surgeons, infectious disease specialists, radiologists, a psychiatrist, research specialists, and so on—were involved in his treatment, not including the psychologist and a dozen nurses.

two

MICHELE'S STORY

Allow me to introduce myself. My name is Michele. I've been cured of leukemia. When I was first asked to talk about this difficult and painful experience, it seemed so simple. Now that I'm about to begin, everything is getting mixed up, vague, and confused. It's even difficult to describe how I feel today. On one hand I'm so happy to have overcome this terrible illness, on the other I'm afraid that death is waiting for me around the next corner. Death, whose company I've shared for so long. I have to convince myself every day that I'm alive and that I'm living a normal peaceful life, a life like anyone else's.

Truly, I don't know where to begin. Should I describe my first visit to the pediatrician? My first admission to Sainte-Justine? Or should I begin with my first treatments, my first injections? I was only a child at the time, four-and-a-half years old. It was in 1964, such a long time ago now. It was a terrible shock for my parents when they first heard the medical verdict. Leukemia. Cancer of the blood. They were very careful not to let their true feelings show in front of me, and they didn't tell me I was seriously ill. I can still hear the doctor's words as he said:

"My little girl, you're going to stay with us for a while. And you're going to play with the other children. It's going to be just like school. Mommy and Daddy will come and visit you and bring you all kinds of beautiful presents. You won't be bored. We're going to take good care of you."

It's difficult now to remember clearly my first stay in the hospital, but these words come back to me easily and often. So I began to play with the other children. I became one of them, sharing their closed world, lovingly watched over by those we naively called "aunty" or "uncle." I adapted easily to my new surroundings, but felt neglected by my parents. They did come to see me, but at that time the rules were quite strict. Visiting hours were always too short and they had to leave as soon as the bell rang. As the precious minutes ticked away I would cry, sob, and beg for them to take me home. I wanted so much to play with my sisters.

I didn't want to be left alone again with these strangers. I dreaded being alone at night. I can still hear my cries and I can imagine the pain they must have caused my mother and father.

I left the hospital a month and a half later, having spent all this time in the company of strangers. Although they had showed me nothing but love and kindness, they had come to represent a threat. After all, I was only four-and-a-half. If they really loved me, why did they stick needles into me? They told me it wouldn't hurt, that it was just like a little mosquito bite, but nothing could have been further from the truth. These well-meaning lies were difficult for a little child to understand. Why were they making me suffer so?

The needles hurt. They hurt so badly that even the thought of getting another one brought on the pain. The mosquito bite, which hardly seemed to bother adults, was for me much more painful than a bee sting. And I'm at a loss to describe those terrible spinal taps. Again the staff lied to me. They said they wouldn't hurt too much.

These very devoted people loved me, however. Looking back, I realize now that several of the nurses gave the impression of being detached from the children in their care. They had to be. They didn't want to get too close for fear of becoming overwrought by the drama of the illness that afflicted us, the little children suffering from leukemia and, in all probability, destined to die very soon.

It's true. Not everyone has the strength to be so close to children who are suffering and in pain. Not everyone has the courage to witness a child's death or the hurt and suffering of the parents, who must stand by helplessly as those they love the most fight for their lives.

It seems that things have changed today, probably because the chances of a cure are much better than ever before. More attention is given to psychological support in addition to the actual medical treatment. A child suffering from leukemia is no longer automatically considered to be living on borrowed time; death is no longer inevitable.

I would be lying if I told you that the first few months of treatment were not painful. I also know that a little girl's imagination can twist the facts and blow things out of proportion to the point where they become unbelievable. I couldn't understand why the doctors had to do so much for a supposed cure that never materialized, at least not so you could notice. Just thinking about them today sends shivers up my spine! During the spinal tap my left leg felt all funny. It made me feel so bad that I even forgot about the pain from the needle in my back. Even today, however, at the age of 22, I shake whenever I hear the words *lumbar puncture*. Please, don't ever talk to me about lumbar punctures!

Not only were the treatments designed to combat the painful leukemia, but the drugs themselves caused unpleasant side effects. If my memory serves me well, I was convinced that those fiendish drugs made me sicker than the sickness itself. I will never forget the side effects from the cortisone and the methotrexate: I turned as pale as a pint of milk and my body became all twisted. That's not so important when you're very young because you're not really too worried about having a beautiful figure or looking like a movie star. But this hideous transformation takes on monstrous proportions when you're approaching fifteen, the age when you know boys are starting to look at you. And these drugs, are they going to have any long-term effects? Are they going to leave scars? If I no longer have a slim waist, is it because of some side effect from those so-called cures? Or am I just being ungrateful? Who can answer me? Only time can.

I'm now studying to become a nurse and, from time to time, I work in the emergency room of a Montreal hospital. I get to see a lot of children who are suffering from leukemia, especially those already receiving treatment. I can spot them because they're the ones who are losing their hair. Their faces are swollen and pale, almost moon-like in appearance. I know that it's the illness and the drugs that transform them so cruelly. I know that they're really beautiful, that they're only temporarily wearing masks.

Among the good memories of the time that I was ill, and believe me there are some good ones, I remember the smiles and greetings of the nurses and the lab technicians. Even today, they still greet me when I visit the hospital. Their warm and friendly welcome makes me believe that I've become important to the staff. I feel good and reassured. They know me, they understand me.

It was not the first hellos that impressed me, but rather those of the last few years, and I've known these people between twelve and fifteen years. They're still kind and thoughtful enough to welcome me with "Hello, Michele. How are you?" and I feel good through and through. I guess I am important to them. After all, haven't they shared a big part of my life? Don't I represent a victory over the illness that surrounds them every day. To each of them I reply, with genuine feeling, "Hello. I feel great, thank you."

I said earlier that I'm training to be a nurse. I would never have the courage to work in pediatrics, though. It would be too painful to watch children suffering. I love children and couldn't bear to hear them crying, "Mommy, Daddy, come and get me." I'd be afraid to feel sorry for them and perhaps indirectly for myself. If I were to see a child die from leukemia, I'd tell myself that it was unfair. I'd rather die instead of the child. And why shouldn't I give my life to save that of another? It's only fate that has allowed me to survive. Or I would tell myself that the child and I had done nothing to deserve being stricken with leukemia. We had not been so bad as to deserve such a punishment. Why did we get it? I'll never be able to answer that question either.

One of the most difficult things to accept, one of the things that had the most profound effect on me was that while I wanted so much to be like other children, I was always treated differently. I was forbidden to run because of the seriousness of my illness; I might hurt myself. At school I could not get into any rough-and-tumble play with my friends; I might hemorrhage. It seemed that I was always waiting.

Waiting until recess was over. Waiting for a crowd of children to pass. Waiting. Because I was always waiting, I came to be afraid of everything. I'd avoid moving and usually ended up sitting alone in a corner, waiting for something that might resemble a normal life. Or perhaps even death, a death without pain. Shyness and timidity became my constant companions. It would have taken only a slight mishap, a little accident to shatter my fragile health and put me right back in the hospital. Even though I've been cured, I live in a world of insecurity, an uncertain, withdrawn world. Oh, I've become used to it. I consider myself to be a calm, collected woman—at least on the outside. Sure, I flare up once in a while, but it takes a lot to make me explode. I believe that I can face up to just about anything. I ask myself whether this is due to the long hours I spent waiting and reflecting during my illness. Did these hours have a decidedly beneficial effect on my character?

I'm what you'd call a stay-at-home. Even at 22, I find it hard to mingle in a crowd. Is this an innate trait, or is it another legacy of my medical past? Nobody knows the answer to that one either. I believe that I have to face the problem alone, like a leukemic child fighting for survival. For no matter what you believe, it's the child who must face up to the awful truth and who must beat the illness. The doctors, nurses and parents are there to support the child and to provide the necessary medical aid, as well as the moral support needed to help achieve victory.

I have to return to the spinal taps. Every time I had one, I had to cope with side effects like nausea, vomiting, and headaches. Whenever it was done by the chief neurosurgeon, as opposed to his assistant, I didn't get as ill. Maybe the procedure was exactly the same. Maybe the assistant could do it just as well, but the unshakable confidence I had in the chief almost completely dispelled any unpleasant after-effects. This serves to show the power of mind over matter. The technical term is *psychism*. It's very powerful and, depending on the individual, can be helpful or harmful.

Personally, I never believed that I would be cured of leukemia. I had seen too many children, who were supposedly cured, suffer a relapse after five or seven years of remission. I used to tell myself "it's been ten years, or fifteen years, Michele, and everything seems to be going fine. People are telling you that you're cured." But that doesn't stop you from always being afraid. Will I have a relapse tomorrow?

A simple illness can become a catastrophe. The anxiety creates a thousand doubts and other symptoms. Has my time come? Perhaps I'm not going to make it this time. Sometimes, I have to consult doctors, not my pediatrician because I'm too old now. I tell them that I once had acute leukemia and that I'm still afraid. Most of them look at me flabbergasted. Then they look skeptical. Then they smile. Surely not this fine, tall woman. Then I explain several medical terms to them and relate specific facts, and they realize that I'm telling the truth. Only then do they take me seriously. I've learned from experience that it's often best not to mention my illness or my past. When the doctor asks me if there has ever been any serious illness in my family, I answer no.

I am cured, aren't I? More and more, I would love to erase the image of the leukemic child that I once was. All of that is behind me, I know, but through my young adult life I want to live a brand new childhood. Oh no, it's not easy to forget the past.

Let me tell you about some of my friends at the time when I really needed someone to talk to and confide in. A few of them stood by me, but most dropped me like a hot potato. Why? Was it because they were simply too busy with other things? I believe that the real reason they drifted away was because they were afraid of being involved with someone who, in all probability, was going to die very soon. When one is young it is difficult to watch a friend suffering and to stay with her to the end. One is too quick to assume the worst, and the slightest illness bolsters this fear. To be young is to be full of life. It doesn't make sense to become attached to someone you believe is getting ready to die.

We live in a world in which only the healthy are respected. Unaware of the nature of my illness, as a child I used to love meeting the other children attending the hematology clinic. When they stopped coming, I would ask my mother where Julie, Mark or Luke were. She answered me, always a little embarrassed, that they had gone to join the baby Jesus. Not only did I lose my friends, but I was sorry that I had ever known them. It hurt to lose friends, the little boys and girls whom I had played with and come to know. I tell myself that this is why some of my healthy friends drifted away. They figured that one day things would take a turn for the worse and that it was better to cut the ties before that day arrived.

There remains one important subject to talk about. Should you tell the truth to a child suffering from leukemia? Should you reveal the nature of their illness to them? In my case, I wasn't told until I was fourteen years old. Ten years had passed since it was first diagnosed, and in all that time I remained in ignorance. Then my doctor told me: "Michele, don't worry about it, it's all part of the past, but you did have leukemia."

How was I supposed to react to this startling news? Cry? Scream? Laugh? I turned quickly to my parents with a questioning look. Surely they could see my disapproval. Why had they kept the truth from me all these years? And my doctor, why didn't he demand that I be told? For a child, the word *leukemia* doesn't carry the same significance as it does for an adult. A child could learn the truth gradually and learn to tame its fears.

When the doctor explained to me that leukemia was a cancer of the blood, I felt very uneasy. The word *cancer* made me tremble. I was aware of the close relationship between cancer and death, and my imagination began to run away with me despite all the assurances the doctor tried to give me. Inside, I couldn't stop telling myself, "Michele, you're going to die. You're going to die." None of the other matters discussed at the time had any meaning for me. I couldn't concentrate on what the doctor was saying. I wanted to cry, to scream. I didn't want to know them anymore, but instead I politely sat in my chair and listened.

The doctor asked me if I had understood everything. I answered yes by nodding my head. I wanted to get out of that place, fast. Oh, how I hated the clinic and, indirectly, everyone associated with it. The doctors and nurses who had been beside me all those years, and whom I trusted, had paid me back by lying to me. My faith and confidence in them had been shattered in a single moment. How could I trust them from now on? Every explanation they now tried to give me would be interpreted as a well-meaning lie. They had lied to me for ten years, why should I believe them now? Were they just telling me this today to prepare me for something more difficult to come? Perhaps I didn't have long to live.

These accusations now seem unfair. That all happened eight years ago, and I've now gone twelve years without treatment. Yet even today the fears come back to haunt me. Fear of another relapse. Fear of death. Fear that I wasn't told the whole truth. I continue to live with fear. Having said that, I must admit that in all probability I have been cured of leukemia. As I grow older, I become wiser and more able to take advantage of the philosophy that life consists of living one day at a time, of enjoying to the fullest everything that it brings.

For this I owe a great deal to my parents, who have lived through this drama since I was a small child. They never complained. They never showed their pain or their worry, and they shared my fear of tomorrow for many, many years. My victory was the reward for their courage and their refusal to give up. For that I thank them.

To all the children now suffering from leukemia, I wish you the same good luck and good fortune.

[Michele is now 26 years old, a nurse, and married; she recently gave birth to a healthy baby girl. —J.D.]

three

SOME STATISTICS

There are those who would like to believe that children are immune to cancer, that it is an illness that only affects adults. It's perfectly understandable why people want to believe that such a terrible affliction would spare those who have not even finished growing up. But this is the brutal truth: cancer strikes more than one in six hundred children between the ages of one and fifteen. This statistic might seem insignificant when your child is one of the healthy ones, but it takes on monstrous proportions when *your* child is stricken. Your child has contracted an illness you always preferred to ignore. It does exist, and it can shatter your life and that of your family.

You have certainly already talked about cancer in your family. There was Uncle James, who smoked like a chimney and who died from lung cancer. There was also Aunt Elizabeth, who passed away from vague "general causes," but given her advanced age you reassured yourself that it was simply a question of old age. Then one of your friends lost her mother, who was quite young, to breast cancer. This disturbed you, for it brought the problem much closer to home.

Then, yesterday, you took your four-year-old son to the doctor. For a few weeks now, he had been tired for no apparent reason, and something strange had appeared on his thigh. You entered the doctor's office convinced that you would leave with a prescription and that all your worries would be over. Then you learned that your son—so active, so full of life—had contracted leukemia. This one word has broken something inside of you. Perhaps you've always taken good health for granted, rather than seeing it as a gift that is given daily. The news has cast you into another world, a world that is completely foreign to the one that you had always imagined your child growing up in.

Every year, thousands of children throughout the world are dealt this cruel blow. In the United States alone, some seven thousand new childhood-cancer cases are detected annually. In Canada, there are almost seven hundred new cases, approximately two hundred of them in the province of Quebec. Some two hundred new cases to treat in addition to the two hundred from last year, and the two hundred from the year before that, and so on. Indeed, the problem is so serious that a provincial hospital such as Sainte-Justine in Montreal receives more than a hundred new cases every year. In addition, it is continually and actively treating about five hundred victims. These patients are adolescents, children, and infants. They come from every class of society and from every region in the province.

Another frightening statistic: for every child, the risk of contracting a malignant tumor (leukemia or another form) before the age of fifteen is approximately .2 percent. This percentage is miniscule when compared to that for adults, which is 22 percent. In effect, the risk of contracting cancer increases with age. The older one gets, however, somehow the less tragic cancer becomes. After all, we must all die some day, and whether we pass on from a heart attack, renal deficiency, or cancer is only of relative importance.

Cancer among children represents only 1 percent of the overall incidence of cancer. This year, of the 655,000 new cases reported in the United States and of the 18,000 in Quebec, 99 percent are represented by adults.

Cancer in adults is very different from that which attacks children, both in terms of form and evolution. Cancer in adults strikes organs such as the skin, the epithelium (giving rise to cancer of the skin), the glandular system, the digestive tube, the lungs, and the liver. These cancers, which are called carcinoma or adenocarcinoma, are for the most part caused by environmental factors. By this I mean known cancer-causing chemicals or other substances with which the victim is frequently in contact. There is also, at times, a certain predisposition to cancer, such as in the occurrence of multiple cancers in a given family, or when cancer strikes individuals who have severe underlying metabolic or genetic disorders.

In the case of childhood cancer, environmental factors play almost no role at all. Less than 10 percent of cases can be even remotely traced back to such factors. It is, therefore, a question of an illness that is somewhat different in form. A new-born baby taking its first breath can have an enormous tumor. Was the child attacked, therefore, while still in the womb? What makes it difficult to answer this question is the simple fact that we still do not know the real cause of cancer.

RISKS OF CANCER	
Among adults	22%
Among children under 18	.02%

DISTRIBUTION OF CANCER
In every 100 cases of cancer, there are 99 adults and 1 child.
In every 100 adult cases of cancer, there are 56 men and 44 women.

INCIDENCE OF CANCER	
Among men:	
Skin	21%
Lung	16%
Prostate	12%
Intestinal, rectal	11%
Urinary tract	10%
Leukemia, Hodgkin's disease	7%
Mouth	6%
Stomach	5%
Other	12%
Among women:	
Breast	25%
Skin	17%
Intestinal, rectal	12%
Uterus, ovaries	11%
Cervical	6%
Leukemia, Hodgkin's disease	6%
Urinary tract	5%
Stomach	3%
Mouth	2%
Other	10%

DISTRIBUTION OF TYPES OF CANCER AMONG CHILDREN	
Of every 100 child cancer cases, the breakdown is as follows:	
Leukemia	35
Cerebral tumours	18
Lymphoma	12
Neuroblastoma	9
Wilm's Tumour	8
Bone sarcoma	5
Rhabdomyosarcoma	3
Retinoblastoma	2.5
Other forms	7.5

Cancer can result from a viral infection associated with factors that favour its growth. A virus, after all, can attack a person at any time, before and after birth. It has been proven that certain viruses can induce malignant tumors in animals or transform normal cells—cells cultivated in a laboratory test tube or dish—into cells that are unquestionably cancerous. In 1972, the U.S. government, under the presidency of Richard Nixon, declared all-out war on cancer. More than $600 million was invested during the first year. The research was directed towards identifying the cause of cancer, as well as to improving the therapeutic weapons with which to fight it. Eighty percent of the budget was devoted to improving means of combatting the illness; 20 percent went directly into research to determine the cause. More than a decade later, the budget of the National Cancer Institute has grown to a billion dollars a year. The greater portion of that budget is now given over to research into the cause of cancer, for the mystery still remains.

What have we learned over the years? We have learned that cancer is far more complex than we had ever thought possible. In fact, it is an illness that seems determined never to give up its secrets. Researchers are fairly certain, however, that it is caused by more than one agent. It seems to be a question of a combination of factors that, when they come together under the right circumstances, provoke disaster. An analogy might be that of the atomic bomb, which must exceed a critical mass in order to explode.

Researchers were rather discouraged. They had never expected such resistance. Many believed that by increasing their efforts ten-fold, by centralizing their research, by developing new techniques, and by using laser beams and the latest in computer technology, they would force cancer to its knees. So far their efforts have largely been in vain.

The more we know about cancer, the more we fear it. It continues to stalk and find victims—more than five million a year throughout the world. Before it, we are almost as powerless as a swimmer who sees a tidal wave surging towards him: by the time he sees it, it is too late to escape. Nevertheless, research continues, with some small steps being made. One day we will wipe this scourge from the face of the earth, just as we did smallpox. We also succeeded in controlling tuberculosis and poliomyelitis (polio). At this moment in time, the battle is against cancer.

I mentioned earlier that childhood cancer differs from adult cancer in cause. It also varies in type. A third of all child-cancer victims have leukemia or cancer of the blood and the blood-forming organ, the bone marrow. The remainder have what we refer to as "solid" tumors. These comprise: cerebral tumors, lymphoma, neuroblastoma, Wilms' tumor, rhabdomyosarcoma, osseous (bony) tumor—such as osteosarcoma and Ewing's tumor—eye tumor (retinoblastoma), and so on.

These tumors are born in deep tissue; that is to say in a muscle, a kidney, or in the brain, among others. Most of them are born in tissue that is, ordinarily, part of tissue said to be *mesodermic* or *embryonic*. Among children, these forms of cancer have a common denominator: in the majority of cases they grow rapidly. This leaves very little time for the doctor to judge the urgency of the case. From the very moment he or she suspects cancer, a thorough investigation must be undertaken. Fortunately, if that is the right word, tumors that evolve rapidly often respond very well to treatment, if it is adequately forthcoming. Each case does demand, however, a clear definition of the type of cancer and the treatment necessary to keep it in check. The cure depends upon these two factors. And I do mean cure, for this is another characteristic that distinguishes childhood cancer from adult cancer: the chances of cure are greater. Indeed, more than 50 percent of children suffering from a cancer believed to be incurable or too advanced in the 1960s are now able to be cured.

One in two are cured today, but that's not good enough. Every child has the right to live, and we are determined to win the battle against childhood cancer.

four

LEUKEMIA

Leukemia, or cancer of the blood and bone marrow, can be defined as a proliferation of cells that have become abnormal and cancerous. As such, and in great numbers (10^{12}), they multiply in various organs, particularly the bone marrow from which the normal blood cells originate (red corpuscles, white corpuscles, and platelets). The leukemic cells become so numerous that they fill the bone cavity, making it almost impossible for healthy cells to develop, and resulting in a dramatic reduction in the number of healthy cells. This imbalance also becomes evident in the peripheral blood, which circulates through the veins. The blood becomes impoverished of healthy cells, resulting in the well-known symptoms associated with leukemia, such as anemia, hemorrhaging, and infection.

Leukemia can be divided into two main groups. There is chronic leukemia, which often occurs among adults but which is practically unknown among children (less than 1 percent of the cases). There is also acute leukemia, which is much more common among young people. Acute leukemia can also be divided into two subgroups: 1) acute lymphoblastic leukemia (ALL), which involves the production of cancerous white cells of the lymphocyte types; and 2) acute non-lymphoblastic leukemia (ANLL), comprising myeloblastic, myelo-monoblastic, monocytic or erythroblastic leukemia, as well as other forms. Here, the leukemic cells are white blood cells that come from the myeloid cell line. Lymphoblastic leukemia accounts for 70 to 80 percent of cases in children, with various forms of non-lymphoblastic leukemia accounting for the balance.

Leukemia usually only reveals itself when the illness is in an advanced stage; a point where a considerable number of leukemic cells have spread, to some extent, throughout the body. For this reason, it would serve little purpose to subject children to blood tests every six months in an attempt to detect the illness before it becomes marked. The work must begin at the moment a child shows an unusual symptom that cannot be otherwise explained. When this happens, the doctor must be extremely vigilant. A word of caution: one should not be too quick in diagnosing leukemia, for there are other benign illnesses—such as infectious mononucleosis—that can resemble it.

Leukemia reveals itself, therefore, when it provokes symptoms. There is no evidence to suggest that it is contagious. It can strike at any age; even a newborn can be attacked. The principal victims, however, are children between the ages of two and five. They generally display the following symptoms:

1. progressive anemia resulting in paleness, fatigue, and a general deterioration in health;
2. a susceptibility to infection leading to bouts of fever that cannot be explained and that are sometimes intense;
3. hemorrhaging resulting in ecchymoses (blue bruises) and purple blemishes, particularly on the lower limbs, but that can appear anywhere on the body;
4. various aches and pains, including aching bones;
5. palpable glands in the neck, the groin, and under the arms, as well as an increase in volume of the liver and the spleen.

These symptoms are the most classic, but the illness sometimes manifests itself in more atypical ways, such as rheumatoid-like arthritis that resists treatment.

In the majority of cases, leukemia is easy to *diagnose*. An examination of the bone marrow can usually confirm the diagnosis. The *treatment* of leukemia is more difficult to determine. One must choose a combination of treatments that offers the best chances for a remission or an eventual cure. The preferred weapon is chemotherapy, accompanied in some cases by cranial radiotherapy. These treatments are painful for the child, particularly during the first three months of induction and consolidation. Once this stage is completed, the maintenance treatment is much easier to bear, even it it must be continued for a period of two to three years. With the exceptions of bone-marrow and spinal taps, these maintenance treatments are not terribly painful; they are more tiresome than anything else.

The chances of obtaining a remission (the macroscopic and miscroscopic disappearance of the illness) are excellent in the case of lymphoblastic leukemia (90 percent) but not as good in other cases (50 to 60 percent). This is also true for the duration of the remission, which can be long in the case of lymphoblastic leukemia, but shorter in other

CHILDHOOD LEUKEMIA			
Group	chronic	acute	
Sub-group	—	lymphoblastic	non-lymphoblastic
Frequency	1%	70–80%	20–30%
Chance of first remission	—	> 90%	50–60%
Average length of first remission	—	3½ years	6–12 months
Average time of survival	—	5 years	9–17 months
Rate of cure	—	40–60%	20–30%

cases. The rate of cure is between 40 and 60 percent for lymphoblastic leukemia, and between 20 and 30 percent for non-lymphoblastic forms of leukemia.

There are charts and information contained elsewhere in this book concerning the advantages and disadvantages of the various treatments. However, one should remember that all of these treatments contain an element of danger. They present both long- and short-term risks. The immediate complications are well known, but the long-term effects have not been so clearly identified. While it would seem *a priori* that there are a few long-term effects, it is important to know exactly what effects the treatment will have on growth, endocrine (hormone-producing) glands, sexual function, and intellectual development. Advancing technology will increasingly enable us to reduce the degree of such secondary effects.

Bone marrow transplants are becoming more and more important in the treatment of leukemia. They are very favourably looked upon in the cases of high-risk leukemias or when a remission occurs after a relapse. It is imperative that the donor be compatible; in other words, the donor must be someone whose tissue is similar to that of the young cancer patient (such as a brother or sister). Special tests enable us to determine whether the donor and the recipient are compatible. Approximately 30 percent of patients can hope to find a compatible donor if they have siblings. A bone-marrow transplant involves anesthetizing the donor and then withdrawing between 300 and 400 cc (cubic centimeters) of marrow through multiple punctures in several bones, such as the pelvis and sternum. This liquified bone marrow is injected intravenously, like a simple blood transfusion, into the cancer victim. Several days before this injection, the patient is prepared for it by receiving intensive chemotherapy and radiotherapy in order to destroy the last leukemic cells as well as his or her own bone marrow, and to suppress the immune system. The liquid marrow of the donor contains young cells that will "populate" the now-empty bone cavities of the patient.

If there is no rejection of the transplanted marrow, this repopulation process will render the patient's new bone marrow fully operational some three weeks after it is introduced. The blood count will stabilize at a normal level, and one can begin to hope that the leukemic cells will not return, that there will be no negative complications as a result of the transplant, such as a serious infection, pneumonia following radiotherapy, or severe graft-vs-host disease. In the majority of cases, this last complication can be controlled by specific medication. A bone-marrow transplant seems simple, but it is difficult for the child who receives it and also for that child's family. All the same, this technique offers an interesting possibility of cure. It could eventually be used in a large number of leukemic children. Studies currently in progress indicate that it might also be possible to use the bone marrow of the leukemic child himself (extracted while the child is in remission) after destroying the remaining leukemic cells by a special technique involving monoclonal antibodies. These antibodies are special substances that are able to detect some specific antigens of the leukemic cells and then to fix on and destroy them. This type of bone marrow transplant should be the ultimate way to cure most leukemic children and will avert most of the complications presently associated with the procedure. But this will not happen in the near future. In the mean time, we have to count on the treatments at hand, mainly chemotherapy. To date, experiments using one of the parents as a bone marrow donor have not been very successful.

After one has obtained a remission, whether by regular treatments or by more radical methods, the major objective is to maintain that remission. A recurrence of the illness—the dreaded relapse—takes the patient back to square one and the future is once more thrown into doubt. The chemotherapy treatment must be more radical. The complications will be more numerous and more serious, and the chances for survival are reduced. Researchers are devoting tremendous efforts to discovering the mechanism by which leukemic cells develop a resistance to drugs. Once this mystery is solved, it will be easy to counter this resistance and to obtain better results.

five

SOLID TUMORS

Solid tumors include all forms of cancer except for leukemia. Their point of origin is an organ or a tissue. When they are first diagnosed, they can be local (restricted to a specific area), they can have spread to surrounding tissue, or they can be linked to metastases some distance away. Surgery is an important weapon against such tumors. One must begin by removing as much of the tumor as possible while avoiding unnecessary mutilation. In the majority of cases, surgery is followed by radiotherapy or chemotherapy, or a combination of the two. For other tumors, however, radiotherapy and chemotherapy play a primary role while surgery is relegated to a secondary one.

There are, generally, eight categories of solid tumors that can affect children. They are:

1. lymphoma: Hodgkin's or non-Hodgkin's;
2. tumors of the central nervous system;
3. neuroblastoma;
4. nephroblastoma or Wilms' tumor;
5. rhabdomyosarcoma;
6. malignant bone tumors;
7. retinoblastoma;
8. other tumors.

LYMPHOMA

A lymphoma is a tumor that is born in the lymphatic glands. There are two distinct families: Hodgkin's and non-Hodgkin's lymphoma.

Hodgkin's Disease

This illness can occur at any stage in life, but becomes more prevalent with age. It's very rare among children under three or four years old and is more common among adolescents or young adults. Another peak period is between the ages of fifty and sixty.

In more than two thirds of cases, the illness manifests itself as swollen glands in the neck or the armpits. Occasionally, it is noticed by the child or the parents, but it is most often detected by a doctor during a routine physical examination. The doctor determines the nature of the tumor according to the characteristics of the mass and its associated symptoms. Hodgkin's disease can also originate in the chest or abdominal glands, where it is more difficult to diagnose.

Symptoms sometimes associated with swelling of the glands caused by Hodgkin's are loss of weight, a high and irregular fever, perspiring at night, and itchiness. These symptoms mainly appear when the illness has reached an advanced stage. The first stages of the illness are characterized by the number of groups of glands that are attacked and also by their distribution. In the most advanced stage, it spreads widely and may be accompanied by metastases to the liver, lungs, bone, and bone marrow.

Hodgkin's disease is usually treated by radiotherapy. In its more advanced stage, one must resort to complex chemotherapy and radiotherapy. The chances of cure are excellent. More than 80 percent of patients suffering from this illness can hope for recovery.

Malign Non-Hodgkin's Lymphoma

Non-Hodgkin's lymphoma among children are malignant tumors, the cells of which derive from lymphocytes. They belong to the same family as lymphoblastic leukemia; the boundary that divides them is actually quite blurred. One could almost consider them to be the same illness but with a different point of origin. Leukemia begins in the stock cells of the bone marrow, while non-Hodgkin's lymphoma begins in the lymph glands.

An early spreading is common in non-Hodgkin's lymphoma and, in more than half of childhood lymphoma cases, the illness has already spread by the time it is diagnosed. Whenever more than 25 percent of the cells in the bone marrow are lymphoma cells, one can justifiably consider the condition to be leucosarcoma or leukemia. This type of lymphoma can strike all age groups, but it is more prevalent from the age of two.

The symptomatology of the lymphoma depends essentially upon the seat (point of origin) of the tumor and the extent to which it has spread. It can include repeated attacks of abdominal pain. It may also include respiratory problems that can threaten the life of the child.

Indeed, this can be the principal symptom. It may all begin with a simple cold, but a thorough examination may discover other clinical signs, and X-rays of the lungs may reveal the presence of a mass there. Multiple abnormal glands in the neck, armpit or groin can also lead to the diagnosis of a lymphoma. Furthermore, common symptoms, such as inexplicable fever, weight loss, loss of appetite, and paleness can be associated with this illness.

In the first stages of a non-Hodgkin's lymphoma, the illness is restricted to one or more groups of glands. In its advanced stage it may attack the bone marrow or the spinal fluid, and sometimes both.

The treatment of a lymphoma is similar in many ways to that of acute lymphoblastic leukemia and comprises primarily polychemotherapy, often associated with radiotherapy directed at the cranial area and sometimes at the areas affected by the tumoral mass. The total period of treatment can vary from one to three years.

The chance of cure among children suffering from non-Hodgkin's lymphoma is practically the same as that for lymphoblastic leukemia. More than 80 percent of the children treated experience a complete remission, and the final rate of long-term response is 50 to 80 percent, depending on how far the tumor has spread at the time of diagnosis.

TUMORS OF THE CENTRAL NERVOUS SYSTEM

Tumors of the central nervous system are born in the brain (cerebral tumors), in the spinal cord (intraspinal tumors), or in the tissues that surround them. These tumors range from benign to extremely malignant. If they are not removed, these tumours are, in most cases, fatal. Two-thirds of cerebral tumors in children are located in the posterior fossa (lower back part) of the skull.

The most common symptoms are as follows: headaches and vomiting—particularly in the morning—neck pain along with a stiffening of the spine, paralysis, seizures, personality changes, and problems with the sphincter muscles, such as the anus.

The diagnosis is made by a neurological examination and by neuroradiological studies. The initial treatment involves surgery. The removal of the tumor is absolutely essential in the majority of cases. It may be followed by radiation directed at the brain and, in some instances, at the spinal column. To date, chemotherapy has only played a palliative role in this condition. The possibility of a remission varies considerably from one patient to another and from one tumor to another.

NEUROBLASTOMA

The neuroblastoma is one of the most common and the most serious tumors among children. The youngsters who are attacked are usually under the age of five. This cancer develops in sympathetic ganglions (the relay organs of the nervous system) or the adrenal gland. The sympathetic ganglions are located on both sides of the spine, from the base of the skull to the point of the coccyx.

This tumor is also often found in the abdomen or in the chest. In more than two-thirds of cases, however, the illness is generalized. The cancerous cells are carried through the blood to the bones and liver, as well as through the lymphatic ducts towards the lymph glands, either close to or distant from the original tumor. A cure can be achieved through surgery if the tumor has not spread, particularly in children under two years of age. For others, this surgery is accompanied by chemotherapy and radiotherapy. One should note that children under the age of one with neuroblastoma—even in an advanced stage—have a better chance of recovery after treatment with chemotherapy (and in some cases with radiotherapy) than older children. Sometimes the tumor will disappear on its own or with only minimal treatment; this, however, is almost a miracle.

The chance of a cure is better if the tumor is not located in the abdomen and if its extension is limited. The chances are not so good if the illness has spread, if the tumor is localized in the abdomen (75 percent of cases are already metastatic at the outset), and if the child is older than one or two. As a result, cure is possible for about one-third of neuroblastoma cases. A period of two-and-a-half years must pass, however, without any evidence of the illness, before a patient can be pronounced cured. Children over the age of two who are suffering from neuroblastoma that has spread to the bone, as revealed by X-rays, have only a 10 to 15 percent chance of cure.

WILMS' TUMOR (NEPHROBLASTOMA)

Wilms' tumor, which originates in the renal tissue (kidneys), is one of the most common among children. Indeed, it represents the most common abdominal tumor in this age group. The tissues of the tumor are similar to those of the normal tissues of the patient's kidney. They are capable, however, of invading surrounding structures and causing metastases to grow at some distance from the tumor, particularly in the lungs. In 5 to 7 percent of cases, the tumor is bilateral, that is, it attacks both kidneys.

Children aged from two to five are particularly susceptible to Wilms' tumor, which is sometimes associated with other malformations, such as the congenital absence of the iris, the overdevelopment of the muscles and limbs on one side of the body, or urinary or genital malformations. The usual symptoms are an abdominal mass, waves of pain in the abdomen and, sometimes, blood in the urine.

In all cases, Wilms' tumor necessitates the removal of the affected kidney. Surgery is usually followed by radiotherapy and chemotherapy for a period of two to fifteen months. Wilms' tumor is highly curable; more than 80 percent of the patients recover fully.

RHABDOMYOSARCOMA

A rhabdomyosarcoma develops in the soft tissues or, to be more precise, in muscular tissue. This malignant tumor can appear anywhere in the muscular fiber, which means in any part of the body. The most common locations are the eyeball, the middle ear, the limbs, the abdomen, and the pelvic region—the vagina, the bladder, and the paratesticular tissue.

As this tumor can be born anywhere, the signs and symptoms can vary considerably. It can cause a tumefaction, such as a swelling of the eyelid, a protrusion of the eye, a lump on the leg, or, if the tumor is in the pelvis, functional problems related to urinating and defecating.

No matter what stage the illness is in or when it is first diagnosed, treatment is dramatic and uses three weapons: surgery, radiotherapy, and chemotherapy. Certain forms of rhabdomyosarcoma are less serious and therefore require less radical treatment. For this reason a rhabdomyosarcoma of the eyeball can be cured by chemotherapy and radiotherapy, thus averting removing the eye.

The possibility of a cure is excellent where a localized form of rhabdomyosarcoma is concerned, and it can exceed 80 percent when the tumor is completely removed. The percentage is decidedly lower when the tumor is in an advanced stage and has created metastases some distance from the tumor. Rhabdomyosarcoma remains a difficult tumor to cure, but the number of children who recover increases every year as the result of a multidisciplinary approach that combines the best of each form of treatment.

MALIGNANT BONE TUMORS

We refer here to tumors developing originally *in* bones and not to the spread *to* the bone of other tumors. Several types of bone cancer exist, but I am only going to deal with two. They are an osteosarcoma and Ewing's tumor. The origins of an osteosarcoma are cells that help to form the bone, while Ewing's tumor is born in the bone, but not, it seems, from the bone cells themselves.

An osteosarcoma is most common among children over ten years old, and it develops most often in the long bones. Ewing's tumor more often that not affects children aged from five to fifteen, and it develops in both the long and flat bones. Both of these cancers can cause a painful swelling of the bone at the site of the tumor. They can also cause metastases to grow quite quickly, particularly in the lungs. The most frequent signs and symptoms are local swelling accompanied by pain.

Treatment varies, depending on whether it is an osteosarcoma or an Ewing's tumor. The approach, however, remains the same. One must treat the primary location of the tumor and prevent metastases. In the case of an osteosarcoma, it is necessary to amputate or, if possible, to simply remove the affected part of the bone. This can then be replaced by a prosthesis, either metal or some other material. Chemotherapy is given before and after this comprehensive surgery. Curative radiotherapy has no place in the treatment of an osteosarcoma. In the case of an Ewing's tumor, on the other hand, surgery plays a completely secondary role. The complete removal of the tumor is recommended when it involves a flat bone, a small bone or, in rare cases, when the tumor is enormous or when, because of its location, other methods of treatment are unlikely to result in a cure. Generally, amputation is rarely necessary; instead, radiotherapy and chemotherapy play a very important role.

The possibility of cure for these two tumors has improved considerably over the past decade. One should remember that less than 5 percent of patients could hope to recover from them in the '60s. Today, some doctors speak of a possibility of cure in 50 percent of cases.

RETINOBLASTOMA

A retinoblastoma is a tumor of the eye that affects babies and small children. The average age of the patients is eighteen months. This tumor is multifocal in that it can develop simultaneously at several spots on the retina of the eye. This means, in many instances, that there are multiple original tumors, a condition not to be confused with metastases. A retinoblastoma can be hereditary. A person who has suffered this form of cancer can, in turn, pass on the illness to half of his or her children.

The great majority of retinoblastoma cases, however, are the result of a new mutation. Nevertheless, whenever one child in a family contracts this tumor, it is wise to have all the children in the family undergo an ophthamological examination. There are two definite signs that can attract the attention of the parents and cause them to seek a diagnosis. One is pupillary reflection and the other a form of strabismus (or crossed eyes). The pupillary reflection, or cat's eye, corresponds to a whitish reflection that can be seen, for example, in a photograph taken with a flash. A diseased eye appears white in the picture, while a normal eye is red.

In the first stages of retinoblastoma, the illness is limited to one or both eyes. When it spreads, metastases can develop as far away as the brain, the bones, and the lungs.

The treatment of retinoblastoma is extremely complex. It is obviously preferable to avoid removing the eye, but this often becomes necessary because of the extent to which the tumor has invaded the structure of the eye. When both eyes are attacked, the most severely affected one is removed, while everything possible is done to save the other and thus the patient's sight. In order to do this, we can resort to radiotherapy, phototherapy, cryosurgery associated with polychemotherapy, and more recently to laser treatment. We are guided by the principle that we must do everything possible to save the child's sight, without ever forgetting that we must above all save the child's life.

The possibility of a cure among infants suffering from a retinoblastoma is better than 90 percent. Our objective now is to obtain a higher level of cure while reducing mutilation as much as possible.

OTHER TUMORS

There are many other tumors that can attack a child, but because of their rarity, I feel they are beyond the scope of this book. I will merely list a few of them: malignant teratoma; tumor of the liver (hepatoblastoma, hepatocarcinoma); sarcoma (fibrosarcoma, histiocytoma); tumor of the endocrine or exocrine glands (ovary, testicle, thyroid, pancreas, suprarenal); and malignant histiocytosis.

six

THE DIAGNOSIS

"Tell me that it's not true, doctor! Tell me I'm dreaming!" a distressed mother pleaded after I had to inform her that her eighteen-month-old son was suffering from leukemia. She rubbed her forehead, trying to drive my words from her mind. For the past twenty-four hours she had been living in fear of hearing them. The day before, her family doctor had examined the child and told her he needed a blood count. She knew that this could mean that her son was merely anemic or that his blood count had dropped, which could indicate something more serious. Now her worst fears had been realized. The hematologist had given his verdict. She cried and sobbed, almost choking on her pain. Her husband didn't say a word. He tried to fight back his tears while looking at the ceiling. He tried not to look at me, giving the impression that he hadn't heard what I had just said. But I knew that my words, such cruel words, had pierced him to the heart. "Tell us that it's not true!"

That same day, I was to repeat this scene with three other couples, telling them that their children's lives were threatened by malignant tumors. Such is the delicate and painful role of a hematologist. You must sit with people who are complete strangers and give them facts that are going to upset and transform their lives.

What is the reaction of the parents or the unfortunate children old enough to understand a little of what is happening? There is no general rule; each reacts in his or her own way. Some arrive at the hospital suspecting that there is something seriously wrong. They are fraught with worry and they want the doctor to tell them that it's a false alarm, that it's only a minor ailment that can be quickly cured with some medication. But the doctor only confirms their worst fears. Others arrive afraid that the little bump they discovered on their child's arm, something that they are first told can easily be removed by surgery, is the sign of something much more serious. We had reassured them, only to tell them later that it was a suspected tumor, and still later, a malignant tumor.

On learning the truth, the majority of parents cry and throw their arms around one another. "It's impossible! Not cancer, not at her age.

And why her? She's never been sick before." After a while, they calm down and ask to know more about the insidious illness that has attacked their child. "Tell us, doctor, will she get better?"

Others have no immediate reaction. Their nerves have already been stretched to breaking. They listen to what you have to say, so frightened that they've been rendered speechless. They don't dare ask any questions. Their reaction, even though it takes a little longer to show, can be equally intense. There was, for example, the father who had been so calm and collected during his meeting with the hematologist. He then got in his car and began to beat on the horn. Alone in his car there was no danger that his sick daughter would see him in such a state. In her presence he was determined to be the unflappable man of steel she thought he was.

Sometimes, a reaction may manifest itself in discord between the parents. The mother may respond impulsively, emotionally. She might sob and cry. The husband, meanwhile, may appear to be a tower of strength, believing he should be strong and in control of his emotions. "Listen to what the doctor is saying or you won't remember anything later." Sometimes the roles are reversed and it is the woman who is the stronger. Ultimately, it's of no importance who is the stronger. Neither role can, here or elsewhere, be attributed exclusively to that of the father or mother. The important thing is that they must support each other. They will be sad, discouraged, and confused. In the hours and days to come, they are going to need each other's strength and understanding, perhaps more than ever before.

In the first few days, the unfortunate parents bombard themselves with questions. They turn to the doctors and nurses and medical staff as if they had all the answers.

"Why is life so cruel to such an innocent child?"

"Why our child? It's not fair. We love her. There are parents who don't want their children, who mistreat them . . ."

"I just can't understand it. My baby has just been born and here I am listening to his death sentence. I can't accept it. If I had known that my baby was going to get cancer, I would never have given birth."

"Surely there's been a mistake. I brought her in with a little bump on her hip, and now you're telling me she has cancer!"

"Why didn't I get cancer instead of my child? At least I've lived. It doesn't make any sense."

"You are going to cure my child, aren't you doctor? You are the specialist."

The doctors listen with all the sympathy in the world. As for answers, they have none. Miracles are not always possible. The doctor can only hope that the parents know they are not alone in this their hour of need.

One must also mention the reaction of children who are old enough to understand what is happening to them, the adolescents and young adults. It is for them that the words *cancer* and *leukemia* take on their full significance. It is they who are setting out on a long and mysterious adventure during which they are, perhaps, going to be asked to give up their ideals, their hopes, and their ambitions. Like young trees that bend in the wind, these youngsters have the strength to come bouncing back, providing one gives them the means and the hope. They are brave enough to fight.

Of course they feel terrible; their physical appearance changes, and they don't have the energy they once had. Still they hang in there, convinced that these setbacks are only temporary and that they're going to be victorious. Sometimes the sacrifices asked of them are great, like missing a school year, losing their hair or, even worse, the amputation of a limb. Despite all the odds, these children want to fight. That's why we believe it is essential to tell them the truth about the nature of the illness and the treatments we propose to give them.

The father of an adolescent told me one day, his voice breaking with emotion, "Tell him the truth, doctor, just as you would your own child." We cannot refuse to accept this responsibility, especially since a child who knows the truth will cooperate more readily with his doctors. In the battle against cancer, the doctor needs his patient just as much as the patient needs him.

seven

COMBATTING CANCER

Have you ever stopped to ask yourself what time means to you? For Alan Watts it is a "kind of movement in one direction going from the past towards the future, through the present."[1] To a certain extent, this definition satisfies the intelligence, but does it represent the concept of time as perceived by each individual? The present, which represents that infinitesimal instant separating the past from the future, is not felt existentially in the same manner by all. One perceives it according to one's concept of the past and how one looks upon the future. The present moment changes second by second to become the past, while flying inexorably towards the future. Should they stop to think about it, it would surely drive anyone searching for permanence to despair. "O time, cease your flight!" wrote the poet Lamartine.

Another definition describes time as continual change, through which the present becomes past. Change is also part of our lives, which are played out in a world in perpetual motion, in constant evolution. Depending on how we perceive change, we establish our own rhythms of living. Some people live at a fast pace, others at a slow one. Every person fights in his or her own way and in the time allotted for some individual goal. For those caught up in a battle for survival, time becomes an obsession.

Children suffering from cancer live in a different time and space. The normal passage of time, from days, to months, to seasons, has stopped for them and for their families. Their time is measured by another yardstick, that of their illness and the stages of its evolution. Like boxers in the arena, they have only a certain amount of time in which to overcome their opponent. The big difference is that the "bouts" have no predetermined length. We are now going to look at the various rounds in this long and difficult fight for survival.

†Translated from *L'Envers du néant*, by Allan Watts. Paris: Denoël/Gonthier, 1978, p. 105.

AN ARSENAL OF THREE WEAPONS

"Yes, the situation is serious, but it's not hopeless. Have faith. We're going to do everything possible to cure your child." Suddenly, when all seems lost, the parents hear the word *cure*. They learn that the battle is far from over and they pull themselves together and show such beautiful determination.

"We'll do it. Charles will get better. My husband and I know he will. We're absolutely convinced of it. You know, doctor, we almost lost him when he was only two months old. He pulled through that time and we know he will again this time. You'll see."

Indeed, few parents today should despair when their child is diagnosed as having cancer. Statistics exist for every illness and they help the doctor to determine the chances of recovery. The figures are very encouraging when one compares them to those of not too long ago. One in every two children is cured. This average does not tell the whole story, however. Some forms of cancer are highly curable. In the case of Wilms' tumor, a malignant kidney cancer, almost 90 percent recover. On the other hand, certain lymphoma and tumors that have already spread when first diagnosed cannot be viewed with the same optimism.

The first stage is critical. It is here that the parents, and the child who is old enough, must take control and face up to the situation. They must understand that the only choice is to fight, to fight with hope, and, equally important, to fight with the will to live. For the battle will be long and hard, demanding energy and superhuman courage every step of the way. There will be no respite until the final victory.

As soon as the particular form of cancer is identified we begin treatment. What is radiotherapy? Will the surgery mutilate the patient? Chemotherapy—doesn't that make the patient more ill than the illness itself? There is so much to learn all at once and this in itself creates confusion. Which treatment comes first? Why begin with one and not the other? Why not go right away to the major medical centres in the United States or Europe? "Of course you realize that we are prepared to make any sacrifice for our child. All we want is for him to get better. Nothing less will satisfy us."

Gradually, the parents calm down. They begin to see things a little more clearly, more realistically. Their questions become more rational. "Tell us everything, even if you think we won't understand what you're saying. We want to know everything that's involved." It is then that the doctor in charge of the case explains all the "weapons" currently used to fight cancer. "In your daughter's case, we are going to resort to three different courses of treatment. First of all surgery, followed by local radiotherapy and intensive chemotherapy. Imagine, if you will, that we are involved in a battle against a powerful enemy.

"Surgery will remove part of the enemy's army. The radiotherapy will bombard those that are camouflaged. The chemotherapy will poison those that have survived the initial attacks and that have had time to leave the battlefield. We have a lot of powerful weapons at our disposal. We need them to fight this sly and deceitful enemy." This is the kind of information and advice the parents get for the moment. They will learn more about each step as the treatment progresses.

Surgery

Surgery has always been particularly popular in the treatment of solid tumors, and we are always hopeful that it alone will give positive results. In the case of leukemia or lymphomas, however, it plays a secondary role, which is essentially diagnostic. Whenever one comes upon a tumor that is visible or tangible, one immediately tries to remove it in the hope that in so doing the illness will be cured. The approach to surgery has changed over the years. At one time, surgeons removed only the tumor and prayed that all would go well. This was followed by a period when surgeons believed in extensive surgery, which often left the patient mutilated. This was done with the best of intentions, however, because they believed it would be more successful. Towards the end of the '60s, they opted for yet another approach. They decided to attack the tumor as much as possible without mutilating the patient.

This approach was made possible by the introduction of two new therapeutic weapons—radiotherapy and chemotherapy—both of which were beginning to enjoy impressive results. The medical profession came to believe that considerable success could be had by combining these two weapons. They were right. In the last decade, the rate of cure has risen to 50 percent for children and 35 percent for adults. Naturally, we are aiming for 100 percent. Other weapons have recently entered the battle, such as immunotherapy and hyperthermia. As yet, they have made no significant impact on the statistics, but they do hold promise for the future. One treatment that is becoming more and more accepted for certain forms of cancer involves delaying surgery and beginning right away with chemotherapy, or using the two combined. The aim is to reduce the mass of the tumor to a point where it becomes easier to remove it surgically some weeks or months later without fear of post-operative complications or excessive mutilation.

It is also important to stress that while surgery plays an important role in certain cases—indeed, it can even lead to a complete cure—it plays a very limited role in the cases of leukemia or lymphomas (Hodgkin's or non-Hodgkin's disease). In these cases it is impossible for the surgeon to remove everything. Chemotherapy or radiotherapy, on the other hand, and sometimes the two combined, will lead to a radical reduction in the tumoral mass or the cancerous cells. They will also make it possible to achieve remissions that can be said to be complete. When we speak of a complete remission we mean that it becomes technically impossible to detect malignant cells in the patient. It should be pointed out, however, that one rarely resorts to surgery for these forms of cancer since the leukemic cells are spread throughout the body. In such cases, chemical agents play a principal role because they can travel through the blood to almost every part of the body. Cranial radiotherapy will reinforce the treatment. On the other hand, a suspect cervical growth will require surgery in order to analyse and define the exact nature of the illness. If it involves a Hodgkin's lymphoma, for example, and if the illness has not spread, radiotherapy will be sufficient to ensure a cure.

Today, the role of the surgeon in the fight against childhood cancer is limited. In the years to come, we hope to take full advantage of new techniques, such as hyperthermia for tumors that are sensitive to heat, and of ultramodern tools such as the laser beam. We also hope most fervently that in ten or twenty years, surgery will serve only to remove tumoral masses, without damaging other parts of the body.

This is already possible with certain forms of bone tumor. After the bad section of the bone is removed, it is replaced with a metal prosthesis or a piece of normal bone. This technique, which is not used very often and then only in specific instances, averts the amputation of a limb. It serves as a model of what we hope to be able to do more frequently in the not-too-distant future. Surgeons have every reason to be proud of the progress achieved to date, but they dream of the day when even more significant contributions will crown their efforts.

They hope that surgery will become even more effective in removing tumors. They also work to improve techniques of cosmetic surgery, which will correct the sometimes less-than-beautiful traces of emergency operations that had to be performed without delay, as in the case of a child whose spinal cord is being compressed by a tumor invading the spinal canal. The slightest delay could cause neurological problems such as paralysis of the lower limbs or the inability to control the anal or vesical sphincter muscles. The child could also experience growth problems at a later date, such as curvature of the spine (scoliosis). Here again, surgery continues to make great strides. Indeed, many children who suffer from scoliosis (either induced or innate) now benefit from advanced techniques that make it possible for them to lead a normal life. Surgeons, always searching for new, improved techniques, will continue to amaze us.

Radiotherapy

Radiotherapy is another technique that we rely on in the treatment of childhood cancer. Formerly known as radium treatment, radiotherapy involves destroying the cancerous cells by directing radiation at them.

Like surgery and chemotherapy, the development of radiotherapy has not always been smooth sailing. It began in 1898 when Marie Curie (1867–1934) discovered the natural radioactivity of radium. In the decades that followed, great progress in the treatment of tumors among both children and adults was made. It progressed from X-rays to gamma rays, and later incorporated neutrons and electrons to become one of the principal weapons in the battle against cancer. Radiotherapy can be likened to surgery in that it has a direct local action on the cancerous cells.

In cases where radical surgery cannot be performed to remove the tumor mass completely, radiotherapy will sometimes be used to destroy any cancerous cells that remain at the surgical site. Its objectives are to attack a metastasis or to destroy a tumor before it has become too advanced. At other times, in the cases of leukemia or lymphoma, radiotherapy will be used as a preventive measure. In such cases it will be directed at the brain and its covering, the meninges, in the hope that it will forestall the problems that often arise with these illnesses: leukemic meningitis and lymphomatous meningitis.

How do these mysterious rays work? The radioactive source is usually incorporated in an impressive machine that resembles a diagnostic X-ray machine but which is bigger in size. This radioactive source emits electromagnetic vibrations that are absorbed by the tumoral cells, thus destroying the tumor. Healthy cells may also be attacked during this process, but they recover much more quickly than the tumoral cells. Before any radiotherapy is undertaken, the tumoral area is clearly defined through various tests and examinations. In effect, a specific target area is mapped out for treatment.

The radiotherapist determines the exact form of treatment after having studied the results of radiography and laboratory tests. With the aid of a computerized tomography (CT) device, the area to be treated is pinpointed and then reference points are marked in red ink on the patient's body. In this way the radiotherapist will be able to apply the treatment in exactly the same area every day for as long as it is required. In general, the treatment is repeated an average of five days a week over a period of three to five weeks, sometimes even longer. Each session lasts only a few minutes. The small red marks defining the field of battle must not be removed at any time during treatment; the delineated area must only be washed with water, never with soap or other cosmetic products. Should the marks fade, the technician treating the child will make sure they are touched up so as to remain visible for the duration of the treatment.

After a few weeks, the area being treated will become a little red, rather like a slight sunburn. This is completely normal. What are the possible side effects? In fact, there aren't many. Sometimes the patient will experience a loss of appetite, which can be accompanied by nausea and vomiting. If treatment is directed at the abdomen it can cause diarrhea; this can be corrected with an appropriate diet and certain kinds of medicine. On the positive side, children are generally much less subject to side effects from radiotherapy than are adults, and thus are better able to undertake this form of treatment.

One should also mention that children receiving treatment in the proximity of the head will experience hair loss. It will grow back, however, when the treatment stops. Before starting any treatment, the radiotherapist will always meet with the child and the parents to explain in detail what is planned. The cooperation of everyone involved is of vital importance.

What is the psychological impact of this course of treatment on the child and the parents? One cannot dismiss this aspect as being unimportant because the very fact that the child is undergoing radiotherapy underlines the seriousness of the situation. Everything is new, unusual, and worrying. Their daily routine has been disturbed. Their morale is low. They often have to change plans that were made some time ago. Parents may even have to juggle their working hours in order to accomodate the medical team. This unknown world can create fear and apprehension. The huge radiotherapy machines, which can appear monstrous, can be extremely disturbing to the uninitiated. Once again, the family has to have confidence in strangers. This, again, can have an effect on the psychological balance of the parents and the child.

It should be remembered that the entire medical team is acutely aware of these problems and that they are willing to do all they can to help the child and the parents get through this difficult period. This is probably a good time to mention the importance of the multidisciplinary approach to the treatment of cancer among children. By this I mean that each case is treated individually; it is presented by a committee or a group to a team of surgeons, hematologists, and radiotherapists. They will discuss each case in detail and decide together when treatment should begin and whether it should involve surgery, radiotherapy, or chemotherapy.

• • •

Paul, aged 12, had a cerebral tumor that the neurosurgeon, as far as he could tell, had removed completely at surgery. Following the operation, Paul received a dose of 6000 rads on his entire brain in order to eliminate any cancerous cells that may have remained. It would be six weeks before this treatment was completed. Paul would certainly lose his hair, but it would grow back in a few months. The neurosurgeon knew that the surgery had been as thorough as possible and that the radiotherapy had destroyed all the remaining tumor cells. He was confident that the tumor would not reappear and that Paul would soon be as alert as ever. He also knew, however, that he would have to watch Paul very closely and examine him periodically with a CAT-Scanner (Computerized Axial Tomography).

Over the next few months, this machine would show that Paul's brain volume had decreased because of the effects of radiation on the support tissue of the brain. This diminution, however, would not overly affect his mental capacity. Paul was in excellent shape and he was intent on doing everything possible to make sure he stayed that way. One could only hope that the CAT-scan would not reveal a recurrence.

Radiotherapy has known some really outstanding successes. I remember a young baby suffering from a bilateral retinoblastoma; both of her eyes had been attacked by cancer. One contained a sizable tumor and was therefore removed. Her other eye, which was less severely affected, had to be saved. The life of this little child was so important to us all. We had to save her. We also wanted to save her sight. For months we tried different forms of treatment, seemingly to no avail. New tumors grew that defied all of our conventional weapons. What could we do? Our only hope lay in a new technique that was being developed in New York. A lot of phone calls were made, paperwork was completed, and the child left for New York. There, a highly specialized team of microsurgeons implanted tiny radioactive metal chips close to the minute tumors. The degree of radiation emitted by these implants was well calculated; it did not extend beyond the area occupied by the tumors. A short time later, the metallic implants were removed. The child is now four years old, and she can see.

Chemotherapy

The third major weapon against cancer is chemotherapy.

"Anything, doctor, but not chemotherapy," cried Elizabeth, aged eighteen.

"Why do you react like that?"

"I don't really know. But I know that it's unbearable. My friend told me one of his parents had chemotherapy. He said it burned. That it made him sick all the time and that, and that . . ."

"And what?"

"And that he lost all his hair. I don't want that to happen to me! No, do anything you have to, but not that."

There's no escaping the fact that chemotherapy has a bad reputation; it strikes fear in all those who hear about it. A lot of people, like Elizabeth, know someone who has gone through it. Indeed, there are currently some three hundred thousand North Americans undergoing chemotherapy treatment.

Because of Elizabeth's reaction, it could have been tempting for the doctor to tell the young girl that some other form of chemotherapy would cure her without making her ill or causing her to lose her hair. Unfortunately, such a treatment does not exist. I truly believe that anyone who discovers a form of chemotherapy that is effective without causing unpleasant side effects deserves to receive the Nobel Prize for medicine not just once, but for several years in a row.

What is chemotherapy? In essence, it involves administering chemical substances either intravenously, in the majority of cases, or orally. These substances are, in a way, a form of poison to the cancer cells. Their role is to attack and destroy these cancerous cells. In doing so, however, they do not always spare healthy cells, giving rise to the disagreeable side effects mentioned above.

Chemotherapy, as we know it today, was not created overnight. It came about over several decades as a result of fortuitous initial discoveries, some welcome additions, and the occasional correction. The first therapeutic breakthrough came around 1942, when military defence studies on toxic gases led to the discovery of a group of chemical substances that were identified as alkylating agents. These agents are capable of bonding the two helixes of the DNA in the nucleus of the cell. If the helixes can't separate, the cell can't multiply, and it therefore dies.

The researchers immediately set about finding a practical application for these alkylate substances. They believed they could be extremely effective in checking the rapid multiplication of cancerous cells. The first results were encouraging. A few years later, in 1947, other studies were made with antifolates, which react against a certain vitamin—folic acid—that is essential for the development of both normal and cancerous cells. Antifolates can induce the most extraordinary results; they are extremely important factors in total remission in the case of acute lymphoblastic leukemia among children. The best known and most widely used antifolate is methotrexate.

The chemotherapy aresenal was subsequently strengthened by a considerable number of other products, including Purinethol and steroid hormones (cortisone). It was discovered that they were considerably more effective when used in combination with other products. This resulted in the emergence of polychemotherapy or combined chemotherapy. This, in turn, gave birth to numerous programs or forms of treatment. Today, chemotherapy has become a very complex weapon. Usually it involves the administration of several drugs, which we hope will lead to more and more positive results with fewer and fewer undesirable side effects.

In the course of the last decade it has become necessary to progress from an empirical approach to a more pure scientific approach. It has also become necessary to discover more about the cancerous cell, particularly its habits and powers of development, multiplication, and defence. This knowledge has enabled us to administer two or three chemical substances that a cancerous cell will readily absorb, even if they are fatal to the cell. For this reason, a better understanding of the cancerous cell has become the primary objective of every research centre. They have returned to the source of the problem; the study of cancer, or rather the cancerous cell, has temporarily taken precedence over the patient. For only when we have beaten the cell, will we be able to wipe out the illness once and for all. That is the ultimate goal: to discover the real causes of cancer and thereby eliminate the disease.

• • •

Maria was suffering from leukemia. Despite the fact that she was barely seven years old, she understood what was happening to her. She was hospitalized—isolated from the other children, as required by her form of treatment. The doctors and nurses were continually giving her injections.

"Why all these needles?" she asked.

"Because we have to use them to give you medicine that's going to cure you."

"But cure me from what?"

"From your illness. You see, the medicine that we give you will chase away the bad cells in your blood, the leukemic cells."

"Why don't you let me swallow my medicine. I'd like that so much better."

What seemed so simple for this little girl is, in fact, a complex problem for the doctor prescribing treatment. Certain drugs can only be administered intravenously (through the veins). If they were taken orally they would be neutralized by stomach acids or enzymes in the intestines. Because of this simple fact, it is not yet possible to change the form of treatment to any great extent. One can only hope that, in time, we will discover new substances that are more specific and less toxic, ones that can be taken orally and that will only destroy the malignant cells.

Vincristine is administered intravenously and can sometimes cause pain in the legs and jaw that may last a few days. Steroid hormones such as prednisone or cortisone will have a profound effect on the child in a few weeks. They can change the child's personality, cause tissue to swell, give the face a moon-like appearance, and stimulate the appetite to the point where all the child can think about is the refrigerator. Fortunately, these changes are only temporary. After the first few weeks, the cortisone is only administered once in a while.

For example, in leukemia, methotrexate is given orally once or twice a week. It can also be administered intravenously or into the spinal fluid. However it is given, it can lead to ulcers in the mouth. 6-Mercaptopurine is a big white pill that has to be taken every day. Like methotrexate and several other drugs, it can reduce the cellular elements of the blood (white cells, red cells, and platelets).

Daunomycin and adriamycin are red-coloured drugs: they frequently cause nausea and inevitably lead to hair loss. There are also mustard gas, Cytosar, cyclophosphamide, thioguanine, L-Asparaginase, actinomycin, procarbazine, bleomycin, cis-platinum, and so on. There are many more drugs that hold out the promise of killing cancer cells. These are just now being tested and have names like 5-AZA-2'-deoxy-cytidine or VM-26.

That is the entire family of chemotherapeutic agents that will crop up again and again in conversations with the hospital staff. Both the children and the parents should familiarize themselves with these drugs; learn to pronounce them correctly, even if they do at first seem like tongue twisters.

Some of these drugs have been around for thirty-five years, but we still don't know everything there is to know about them. Can we refine these drugs even further in order to make them more tolerable for the patients? Can we extract the most active molecules from them and then increase the dosage while reducing the unpleasant side effects? Can we modify them to the point where, with the aid of computers, we can create the ideal drug, the base of which would contain the active elements of each of these substances? Perhaps we can even take full advantage of the drugs by administering them in super doses. This treatment involves giving intravenous medication in doses that are potentially fatal; they are followed some hours later by the injection of an antidote, thereby saving the patient from death while holding out the promise of complete recovery.

This new form of treatment has been explored during the past five to ten years. For example, in the case of an osteosarcoma (bone tumor), very strong doses of methotrexate are administered over a period of a few hours. If the patient does not subsequently receive the vitamin that is the antidote, the results are disastrous. In the following days the patient would suffer atrocious burns at all mucous levels—in the mouth, the intestine and the bladder. A terrible death would ensue. But none of this happens because the folinic acid prevents it, as well as saving the normal cells. This type of treatment is still in its early stages, but it may become more widely used, particularly if we can come up with a drug that will attack the abnormal cells in a more specific manner.

A leukemic child does not receive the same treatment as a child suffering from a brain tumor. And a child suffering from a brain tumor does not receive the same treatment as a child suffering from a neuroblastoma or a Wilms' tumor. Experience gained over the years has enabled us to determine the appropriate form of treatment for each specific cancer in terms of the nature of the illness, its growth, and the stage of its development.

Let's look at the protocol or schedule determining the treatment prescribed for Helene, an eight-year-old leukemic patient. It is one of the most commonly used and also one of the most effective. In the course of treatment, Helene had to pass through three distinct phases. The first was the induction stage, at the end of which we had to obtain a remission. The second stage was one of consolidation. The third was one of maintenance, which in Helene's case could last two to three years. If after all this time Helene is still in remission, the treatment will be discontinued. She will have to remain under medical observation for a few more years, however, so that her cure can be definitely confirmed.

The three months of treatment during the induction and consolidation phases were painful. Over the course of three weeks, Helene received numerous injections, two or three bone-marrow punctures, six lumbar punctures, and cranial radiotherapy. In addition to this she had to cope with noticeable physical changes that were both emotionally and physically upsetting. She often felt nauseous, at times she gained excess weight and fluids, and she lost her hair. Once past the induction and consolidation period, things got a little easier. All she had to do was take some pills and have an intravenous injection once a month. She resumed her normal activities. The nausea passed, the extra weight and fluids disappeared, and her hair grew back. At first her hair was a little darker and curlier than before she began treatment, but towards the end of the first year it regained its former colour and texture.

• • •

Sophie, aged thirteen, did not have leukemia, but she did have a malignant bone tumor, an osteosarcoma. Her first experience with the medical team was a dramatic one, to say the least. The upper leg bone had been so badly attacked by the tumor that her leg had to be amputated. Sophie would never be able to forgive the people who had subjected her to such a terrible mutilation. The treatment that followed was also very painful. She had to undergo chemotherapy four or five days a month for quite a long time. She also had to take strong doses of methotrexate followed by the antidote, as well as adriamycin. These were miserable days for Sophie. She was nauseous and vomited continually, despite all the medical and medicinal support she received from the staff.

"Doctor, why are you giving me this horrible stuff? You've already taken away my bad leg. Why do I have to be tortured for another year? I won't be able to get through it."

"We want to cure you completely, Sophie. The tumor that made you ill has a nasty habit of causing malignant cells to grow in the lungs. So far, we haven't found anything in your lungs. That's a good sign, but we know from past experience that these tiny cells can still exist, and we want to eliminate them. This means we have to rely on drugs."

Sophie asked the same question over and over again, and every time she received the same answer. She suffered a lot, but she soon came to understand that she was not alone and that the medical staff would do everything they could to make the procedures as painless as possible.

Several young patients would have experiences similar to that of Sophie. In each case, we would resort to the same three weapons. The form of chemotherapy might vary, but each would have a name like VAC, POMP, ABVD, or MOPP. These letters stand for known drugs administered according to a pre-established program. For a better understanding of how one of these protocols is scheduled, see the chart on page 58.

The parents hope each treatment will produce the miracle that will cure their child. Unfortunately, doctors are not in a position to promise them anything. A spectacular remission can lead them to believe in miracles, only to have their faith shattered by a dramatic relapse just when everything seemed to be going so well.

There are still so many facets of the illness that are mysteries to the medical profession. The clinical facts are well known to us. But in matters relating to the nature of the illness, particularly its origins and causes, we can only make hypotheses that may be confirmed some time in the future. Whenever doctors quote statistics, they are in fact underlining the impotence of existing drugs. When they talk of a 50 percent cure for childhood cancer patients, they are admitting that known drugs are incapable of helping the other 50 percent. They are powerless against an enemy that so far has revealed only half of its secrets. We must clear up the remaining mysteries if we are to eradicate cancer. It is war, and the front-line troops are the doctors specializing in cancer and the researchers involved in the study of cancer. In my opinion, it would be absurd to give any other group this awesome role.

There are many sellers of false hope, quacks and charlatans who hover like vultures around cancer victims and their families. You just can't imagine how many solicitations these families recieve. They are told "in confidence" during an anonymous phone call: "Don't go see your doctor. He'll only make your child sicker. They're only working for profit.

The ALL Protocol
used in a case of acute lymphoblastic leukemia*

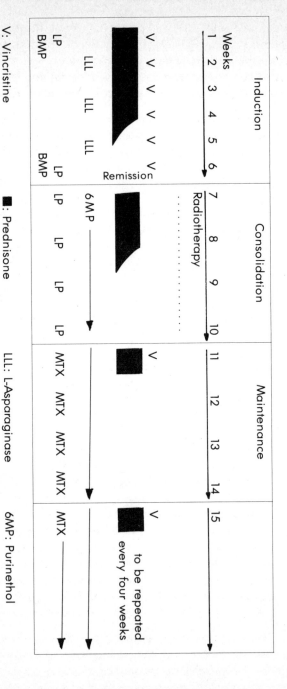

V: Vincristine

LP: lumbar puncture with
   intraspinal MTX

MTX: methotrexate given
   orally once a week

*This is just one example; several other protocols may be used.

■ : Prednisone

BMP: bone marrow
   puncture

LLL: L-Asparaginase

6MP: Purinethol

They're more interested in protecting their monopoly and in making money than in curing your child. Even some pharmaceutical companies are in on the act—in a very discreet way, of course. Come and see us. We'll give you some products that will make you feel well and that will, with the help of your own resources, cure you of this terrible disease."

These supposedly miraculous products go by various names. The best known are Laetrile (an apricot extract) and Essiac (a "magical potion" derived from wild plants). The mysterious formula for Essiac, it seems, was given by an American Indian to a Canadian nurse, who has been using it for years. There is also the Donatian method, imported from Mexico, which involves simultaneously giving insulin and chemotherapy agents. There is also a therapy proposed by healers from the Philippines. Then there is the black market in Interferon; each capsule sells for the modest price of $50,000. The worst thing, however, is that Interferon—which can be found, incidentally, either in negligible quantities or not at all in the "magic" pill—may only be effective when it is administered in a sizable dose and even then only in a few cases. And then only if given intravenously, and so on.

One day, while I was working in a hospital in California, I noticed that the parents of a young 12-year-old girl whom I had been treating for Hodgkin's disease, suddenly became extremely aggressive. Up until that time, our relationship had been excellent. Sophia had undergone chemotherapy and radiotherapy without too many problems. Of course, she hardly enjoyed the experience, but the last six weeks had passed without any major crisis. So why this sudden about-face? Why did I feel the father was being hostile towards me?

"Doctor, you haven't told me the truth."

"I don't understand why you're saying that."

"You understand me, all right. Friends have told me that my daughter will become deformed like a mongoloid. That she'll no longer be able to lead a normal life."

"Excuse me, but I've told you everything about her illness and the treatments we're giving her. We explained they would cause certain unpleasant side effects. The things you're describing haven't happened to your daughter, so who put these ideas into your head?"

The man refused to tell me anything more. That same day, Sophia completed the first part of her usual treatment and left the hospital with her father. I could not believe what I had heard, but still I felt sure they would return the following week for the second part of the therapy. They did come, but there was no change in the father's attitude.

"Sir, now it's your turn to tell the truth. Be honest with me. I know that you adore your little girl, . . ."

He began to cry, not daring to look me in the face. And then he said:

"You know that I am Mexican—"

"Ah, I understand. People are putting pressure on you to go to Mexico."

He looked at me in astonishment. How could I possibly know that people had proposed he invest in Laetrile treatment? He had not dared mention it to me for fear that I would be angry at his lack of confidence in me and that I would react badly, perhaps by treating his daughter with animosity or indifference.

"Don't be upset. I'll tell you everything I know about this drug. And then you and your family can decide whether you want to go back to Mexico. And please don't think that I'm going to treat you any differently now than before. All I'm interested in is treating your child the best way I can so that she can be cured. The rest doesn't really matter. But you should know right away that you're not the first to be confronted with this dilemma. Almost all of the cancer patients in this part of California, particularly those of Mexican origin, have been solicited one way or another. People who don't even dare to give their names claim that any young cancer patient being treated here is a plaything in the hands of the doctors, and that the children will turn into hideous, abnormal monsters."

I then proceeded to explain very clearly all that I knew about this so-called medication, which goes by various names, as though those who advocate its use are deliberately trying to make it even more mysterious.

Laetrile, or Amygdaline, or Aprikern, is an apricot extract. The only definable substance that it contains is cyanide. The origin of this so-called medicine goes back to 1920 in California, when a Dr. Ernest Krebs Sr. tried to improve the taste of bottled whiskey by adding apricot seeds to it. The result, according to him, was a substance with medicinal properties. His son, also a doctor, continued in his father's footsteps, and in 1952 he announced to the world that he had extracted a substance that was going to revolutionize the treatment of cancer. In the decades that followed, a monumental fraud saw this substance generate millions of dollars for its promoters. It continues to do so today. This treatment is based on diverse theories, including that of a Scottish embryologist by the name of John Beard. Beard was of the opinion that cancer is a single illness resulting from an aberration of the trophoblastic cells. He therefore concluded that all forms of cancer would respond to one form of treatment. This led him to propose that a single substance was adequate for the treatment of cancer patients. That substance was cyanide, obtained from cyanogenic glucosides, hence Laetrile.

The promoters of Laetrile even had the audacity to name their product Vitamin B-17, knowing that the magical word *vitamin* would carry more weight with the public. *The therapeutic effects of this drug are nil.* This has been confirmed through numerous tests by the National Cancer Institute and the Sloan-Kettering Memorial Hospital, both in the U.S.A. Public opinion and pressure have recently led to further investigations. The conclusions remain the same. As for its effectiveness as a vitamin, this is also unsubstantiated.

Those who defend cyanide have pointed to the Hunzas, who live in a remote part of the Himalayas. The Hunzas, it was claimed, live for an exceptionally long time and illness is virtually unknown among them. Their diet includes a lot of food based on apricot seeds. A Japanese expedition visited the Hunzas and to its amazement discovered a people who were badly nourished and who suffered from a great variety of illnesses, including cancer. The sellers of Laetrile were far from discouraged, however, and came out with another preposterous claim. This "vitamin," it seemed, was now capable of *preventing* cancer. What a magnificent way of exploiting the phobia of cancer that is so prevalent in North America.

Let us return to Sophia and her father. The very fact that we, the doctors who were treating his child, knew about this form of treatment, comforted him. He left that day convinced that we were allies once again. Sophia returned the following month for her last treatment. She was beautiful and happy, and her father brought her to us confidently and in complete peace of mind.

Essiac has also known some popularity in our part of the world, thanks to newspaper and magazine articles. Here, once again, we hear of a plot by the medical profession to keep this "medicine" out of the reach of those who could benefit from it. Because of public pressure, a Canadian university was allowed to use it in their clinic without it first being subjected to all the studies and tests normally required for a new drug. It should be pointed out that before being administered to humans, a drug must first be scrupulously studied *in vitro* (in the test tube) and used in experimental tests on animals. If it is then considered to be sufficiently effective it can be administered experimentally, but only under clearly defined conditions and strict controls. It generally takes five to ten years before these steps are completed. Enormous precautions are taken and only the most effective and safest of drugs ever find their way into the clinic. To give you a small idea of the organization that this requires, almost ten thousand new products or drugs are submitted annually to the National Cancer Institute in the United States. Of this number, only two or three are eventually accepted. The others are refused because they have not been sufficiently studied or tested, because they are of little importance, too toxic, or inferior to substances already in use.

Laetrile failed the test when it was recently submitted. Essiac, which was used in the Canadian clinic without having been submitted, was found to be totally ineffective. After having used it without success on several cancer patients, all of whom were volunteers, the medical team, which had more or less been forced into trying Essiac, gave it up as a dead loss.

One must have confidence in the officially sanctioned medicines. Despite their imperfections, these drugs have evolved from serious research undertaken by the major hospitals, universities, specialized institutions, and the established pharmaceutical laboratories throughout the world. It is inconceivable that the men and women engaged in this research are involved in some kind of devious international plot. It is inconceivable that, either out of professional pride or greed, they would obstruct the introduction of a treatment that could contribute to the cure of cancer. Anyone who does believe this is suffering from an acute case of mythomania. However, having confidence in the legitimate medical profession is not sufficient in itself. One must also support the doctors and researchers, providing them with the means to continue their studies. The state cannot assume the total cost of their research, and the generosity of individuals is therefore always welcome.

However, medicine, with all its resources, cannot do everything. The role of the parents is of primary importance in the overall treatment. Nothing can be achieved unless they are fully involved. The Americans have defined a certain method of treatment as "holistic"; support given a patient is broken down into three categories: physical, nutritive, and moral. The parents play a leading role in this approach to treatment. There are many mothers and fathers who believe, and in all probability rightly so, that their own moral strength can come to the aid of their child.

In her book, *Mona*, Ginette Bureau speaks eloquently of the role of the parents. The author speaks from experience because her own daughter was stricken with leukemia. She truly believes that her own inner strength and determination helped Mona.

Ginette Bureau is not alone in her beliefs. Indeed, studies are currently underway in the U.S.A. to determine the impact of such a global approach on the evolution of an illness. The research is also attempting to determine whether religious faith and the way in which it is practised is in any way related to a cure. I am partial to any approach where inner resources come into play, even though I have no tangible proof that they are effective. Above all, I remain convinced of the inestimable value of anything that can be done to give medicine a warmer, more human aspect.

● ● ●

Amelia was upset. Despite her tender age of seven months, she seemed to understand that she was terribly ill. Many parents have reported that much to their amazement, it appeared that their infant children had a grasp on what was happening to them.

Amelia's stomach, which had been operated on, was hurting. No, Amelia was not happy at all. She made a face. Her big eyes darted from one corner of the room to the other. They were not the soft, gentle eyes that her mother loved. "What's the matter, Amelia? Are you tired?" she asked.

No reply. Amelia had decided to remain silent and to ignore this hostile world around her. Her mother leaned over the fragile little body and took Amelia's face in her hands. She sought her daughter's eyes, trying to arouse her with her voice.

"Amelia, it's time that Mummy talked to you as if we were two grownups, two good friends. Amelia, look at me. I know that you're sick. The surgery has mutilated you, and the disease continues to eat away at the little hope we have left. You must get better. But to do that, you're going to have to fight. Mummy will give you all her love and all the energy she has left. And together we'll win. We'll beat this thing, and you'll be well again."

Amelia looked at her mother and seemed to understand. Her eyes sparkled and her little hand reached out to touch her mother's hair. The world was fine once again. Together they would fight Amelia's cancer of the liver until the battle was won, no matter how long it took. Nothing could come between them, and nothing would cause them to lose faith.

THE THREE WEAPONS			
	Surgery	Radiotherapy	Chemotherapy
Leukemia	—*	+	+++
Lymphoma	±	++	+++
Hodgkin's disease	±	+++	+++
Cerebral tumour	+++	++	—
Neuroblastoma	++	++	++
Wilms' tumour	+++	+	+++
Osteosarcoma	+++	—	+++
Ewing's tumour	+	+++	+++
Rhabdomysarcoma	++	++	++
Retinoblastoma	+++	++	±

*The symbols + and — indicate the degree of reliance on one of the three weapons for each category of cancer. The dash indicates that this form of treatment is not used or is not really effective.

SIDE EFFECTS FROM COMBINED TREATMENT

Handicaps as a result of having limbs amputated or organs removed.
Loss of hair.
Nausea and vomiting, constipation or diarrhea.
Drop in blood count with the possibility of secondary infections, anemia, and hemorrhaging.
Tiredness, general weakness,.
Pain.
Burning sensations, sometimes there are burns in the areas that have been injected.
Psychological problems.
Long-term effects (rare) include deformity, atrophy, and another cancer.

N.B.: While all of the above listed side effects are possible, a patient will not necessarily experience all of them.

eight

THE REMISSION

ONE MOTHER'S VIEW

"It's so painful being the mother of a child who has cancer. My seven-year-old son has had leukemia since the age of three. Perhaps he is cured. How can we tell? I don't feel I have the right to complain, because I have hope. Even so, I would like to explain some of the things that still torment me.

"In the beginning—it seems so long ago now that the memories are blurred—there was the shock, the anguish, the storm. I had to pull myself together, to stop thinking about it, to live one day at a time. Above all we had to pull Patrick through before he became too marked by the experience. There were several people taking care of him, a mother, a nurse, a psychologist, and other professionals; what he didn't need was a wounded woman.

"I hid my suffering from him. I talked to him about his problems, not mine. That's normal, isn't it? But I suddenly realized that my son thought his leukemia didn't affect me. How could anyone be so wrong. I cried and he was reassured that I loved him. I love him so much. I realize now that Patrick doesn't need a perfect mother, he needs one who is human.

"Yes, I'm afraid, terribly afraid that Patrick will get sick again. Yes, I love him, and I will give him everything that I can to avoid another illness. I know that I'll never be able to stop worrying about his health, his life. I also know that I should be thrilled that the first battle is almost won. I'll be so happy when I can stop giving him all those drugs. But I'm afraid, very afraid. Sometimes I get so anxious about what can happen next that all my worries come flooding back, worries that I've never really expressed but that are always there.

"Yes, I'm enraged. I just can't bear to watch children suffer. Not only Patrick, but all children. Every time I see their brave little faces, it hurts. But what can I do with all this anger? It makes me sick.

"Yes, I feel guilty, guilty as hell. There are times when I feel like apologizing to Patrick. I want to ask him to forgive me for having given him such a fragile existence. But I've never regretted his being born. I'm so happy to know him and to love him. He's full of laughter, you know, full of life. He has lots of friends. He's always asking questions. He gives me his tenderness, his charm, his fantasies, his humour and his seriousness, his life. We love each other and, through him, I've learned to enjoy life minute by minute.

"I have a husband and another son, whom I love just as much and who bring me great happiness. But it is a different kind of love in that there's no feeling that it might all end soon. It's not as fragile as the love I feel for Patrick. With him, my moments of happiness are tinged with sadness. They're so intense, though, that they're worth every second we share.

"Yes, it's hard to be Patrick's mother, but it's also a great blessing, and a great joy."[1]

Michèle Laverdure D. could not have expressed more clearly how parents feel when their cancerous child is in remission. Despite the passage of time, this woman, the mother of a leukemic child who is progressing normally still asks herself many questions. Did she dream it all? No. She wishes that the sword of Damoclese could be removed from over her son's head. The doctor can't confirm anything for the moment. The treatment is drawing to a close and Patrick has beaten all the odds quoted by the doctor at the first examination. Is he really on the road to recovery or is the illness just playing tricks, giving rise to false hope?

Even though there is every chance that Patrick is now cured, his parents probably won't ever be convinced of the fact. It's not easy to live through this period of remission, plagued as it is by questions and doubts.

While some leukemic children in remission can live a relatively trouble-free life, able to do just about anything they want, others who have undergone more rigorous chemotherapy will experience unpleasant side effects and have a rougher time of it in general. The nausea and vomiting caused by the injections can become unbearable nightmares that, in some cases, seem even worse than the illness itself. For some parents the solution is obvious: "Doctor, our child is well. It's been over a year since he was treated for leukemia. What point is there in continuing? We're convinced that he's cured. Do some tests and you'll see that he's just fine."

[1] Michèle Laverdure D., published in *Information Leucan*, XII, 4, oct-nov-dec 1981, p.3

We hear this request all the time. In some cases, the parents will even decide to discontinue treatment and look for assurance elsewhere. They may turn to so-called natural products or to charlatans of all kinds. Doctors repeat over and over again that even though no signs of the illness can be detected, this does not necessarily mean that the patient is totally cured. It's always possible that a few malignant cells have escaped the intensive treatment to survive in microscopic quantities. If they do exist, there is always the possibility that they will multiply, causing a recurrence or a relapse in a few months or even a few years.

Recurrence and *relapse*. These two words can poison the period of remission and give rise to enduring fears.

- Fear that the illness is only sleeping and that any day it will awake.
- Fear of the slightest change in the blood count: "Tell me, doctor, why aren't there enough granulocytes and platelets in the blood? Why the word *meta* here? Does that mean metastasis? This new bone marrow, isn't that proof?"
- Fear of a swollen stomach: "Maybe he just ate too much last night."
- And the splitting headache? "Perhaps it's nothing. I get them sometimes. Maybe it's linked to her sinusitis. What if it's the first sign of leukemic meningitis?"
- Fear of a slight fever: "His brother has a cold. There's probably nothing more serious than that wrong with him. But we'd better call the doctor to be on the safe side."
- "Why has she got ulcers in her mouth? And why isn't she running around like she usually does. She's hardly eaten anything in the last couple of days. Why has she lost her appetite?"
- "Why does his leg hurt this evening? He had the same problem when the doctor first . . ."
- "I'm scared to send her to school. She needs to be protected no matter what the doctor says."
- Fear of the attitude of the doctor during the last visit to the clinic: "Why did he look that way when he examined Yannick's stomach? Why did he take so long to study the X-rays?"
- "Why is she starting to lose her hair again, just like that, for no apparent reason?"
- "He's our only child. That's why we're even more concerned. Oh, we know we shouldn't be so protective. The psychologist explained it to us, but that doesn't make us any less afraid."
- "And chickenpox. We don't even want to think about it. Yet

in all the literature and pamphlets we've read it says that chickenpox can attack children whose defences have been weakened by chemotherapy. In some case, it can even be fatal, but what can we do?"

At this stage, the doctor should clarify certain points with the worried parents and their children in order to reassure and comfort them as much as honestly possible. The first phase is over and with it, the majority of complications. The child should now feel relatively good and should begin to feel like any other child.

Unfortunately, some children never reach this stage. They have known only problems and complications from the start. The end comes without them ever having enjoyed a respite, without ever having experienced a remission. However, more than 90 percent of the patients suffering from acute lymphoblastic leukemia will experience a remission that lasts, on average, more than three and a half years. On the other hand, only 50 to 60 percent of the patients suffering from acute myeloblastic leukemia will experience a remission lasting, on average, 18 to 24 months. Almost all the children with a solid tumor react favourably to treatment and will know a period of respite. It is in this group that we see the greatest percentage of cure. In all instances, however, the period of remission is frequently linked to a big question mark, and the parents continually ask themselves whether their child will be one of those who pulls through.

The chart on page 69 illustrates what actually happened to a five-year-old with acute leukemia. When the illness was first diagnosed, the whole organism, and particularly the bone marrow of the child, was already stricken with leukemic cells. They numbered about 10^{12} (a trillion). If one could compress these billions of cells into a container, they would equal a mass of one kilogram. They are so powerful and they occupy such strategic positions in the body that they weaken the organs. In doing so they create a host of secondary problems; they can even cause death. From the moment treatment begins, these malignant cells begin to decrease in number. After one or two months, at the time of the full remission, their number has dropped to 10^9 (a billion). Their weight would now equal one gram. They are, therefore, a thousand times less numerous than before. These cells are still hidden throughout the body, though, and it is impossible to detect them all, even with a bone-marrow puncture.

At this point, the doctor can begin to talk of a remission, despite the fact that some malignant cells remain. Chemotherapy and radiotherapy over the next few years will either completely eliminate

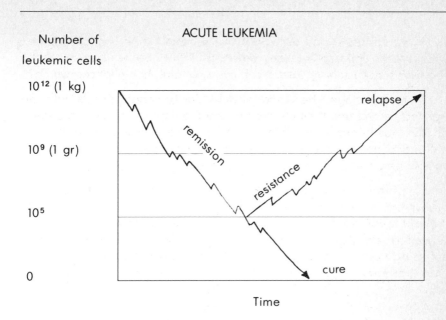

Number of leukemic cells

10^{12} (1 kg)

10^9 (1 gr)

10^5

0

remission

resistance

relapse

cure

Time

them or reduce their strength to 10^5 (100,000). These one hundred thousand cells represent a mass smaller than the tip of a fine ballpoint pen. In all probability, the body itself will be able to eliminate them with its own defence systems and immunological mechanisms. It is not until these last leukemic cells have disappeared that we can possibly talk of a patient being cured.

Unfortunately, there is as yet no test sophisticated enough to determine whether any malignant cells remain. Doctors therefore rely on past experience, confirmed by statistics, and hope that time will prove them right. They do go to great lengths, however, to make sure that all the odds are in their favour. Discontinuing chemotherapy too early on in the case of acute lymphoblastic leukemia, for example, can render the patient susceptible to a relapse.

This uncertainty over whether malignant cells remain is a cause of great concern for everyone involved. Is the patient really cured, or are there still malignant cells somewhere, oscillating between 10^5 and 10^9 in number? Studies and new tests are currently being conducted that will perhaps enable us to detect these remaining cancer cells or even a relapse a few months before it becomes clinically apparent. But these studies don't provide all the answers. For example, why don't some of the cells respond completely to treatment? Why do some persist, reappearing in the bone marrow and in the blood? How do they build up resistance to treatment? This resistance is the primary cause of a relapse, and it is imperative that we learn more about the complete mechanism of the cell if we are ever to beat it.

Research teams, including ours at Sainte-Justine Hospital, are working all-out to find the answers to these perplexing questions. If we are successful, we will have made a giant step towards resolving the tragedy of leukemia and of cancer in general.

The years of waiting and uncertainty have different effects on the families involved. One family can only think of the end of this terrible experience. Another lives only for the treatment in progress. Still another wraps the child in a protective blanket, forbidding him or her to become involved in all sorts of activities for fear of upsetting some delicate balance. Some children are even kept home from school.

A large number of parents do try, however, to live one day at a time, enjoying the good moments, and accepting the uncertainty of the future. They don't always succeed, because anxiety is a tyrant that is not easily overthrown. Nevertheless, they philosophically manage to accept the moments of happiness and joy that life can bring.

During this period of remission, families must face other challenges. They must put themselves out on numerous occasions, they must be prepared to change their routines. They might even face financial problems. Above all, they must learn to accept the painful reality of treatment, not only with regard to injections and punctures, but also the side effects that might arise from them. For example, the burns on a hand because some drops of medicine were injected outside the vein. Or a bleeding irritation of the bladder, rare but extremely painful. Incidents like these are a source suffering for the young patients, as well as of worry and uncertainty for the parents.

Sometimes it's all too much for the children. They get tired easily and feel worn out. They will vomit for days at a time. Some children show symptoms of unpleasant secondary effects even before they receive the medication. Peter was a case in point. We could hear him crying as soon as he entered the building, and we were on the third floor. He only calmed down on the fifth and last day of each treatment session. The same drama was played out every month. This "torture" lasted for two years. Today when he visits the clinic, it is an entirely different story; he is all smiles and the staff greet him like an old friend.

Sometimes the situation can become unbearable. One 17-year-old girl, suffering from a bone tumor, decided that she had had enough and that she would discontinue treatment. She described it as being "worse than hell." We could only hope that fate would be kind to her.

One of the real problems that can arise during this period of remission is the unforeseen infection that, independent of the illness itself, can complicate matters and throw everyone off track. Some of the most frequent infections are viral hepatitis, pneumonia leading to a parasitic infection (pneumocystis carinii), and chickenpox. This last is usually a benign childhood illness, but it can become particularly malicious in the case of a young leukemic child who is undergoing treatment.

● ● ●

Stephanie, a charming young girl of seven, had been suffering from leukemia for three years. All was going well until one day her mother noticed blisters on her daughter's skin; they could only mean one thing—chickenpox—so she contacted the doctor immediately. A few hours later, Stephanie complained of pains in her back and stomach. The blisters were spreading and becoming larger. She was admitted to the hospital for a complete check-up and treatment. In the middle of the night she went into convulsions. X-rays showed that the chickenpox had attacked her lungs. We feared the worst. Because of the seriousness of the situation, the doctor called in all the help possible—infectious disease and lung disease specialists, as well as pediatricians specializing in intensive care. With the approval of the hematologists, it was decided to give her Acyclovir, an antiviral drug that was then still in the experimental stage.

After the first dose, Stephanie's condition continued to deteriorate and she became more and more dyspneic. She could hardly breathe and all her tissues were lacking oxygen. What to do? It was decided to give her oxygen directly. The anesthetist asked to insert a respiratory tube in order to have greater control over the level of oxygen, but Stephanie could not tolerate the tube, which was inserted into her trachea. It was necessary to curarize her—to paralyze her—so that she could not react physically to the irritation caused by the tube. The stress was becoming too much for her. The blisters covering her skin had rendered her almost unrecognizable. Her blocked lungs couldn't draw the oxygen she needed to survive. Her parents were becoming more and more anxious. Stephanie no longer showed any signs of leukemia, but was she now going to die from chickenpox? They refused to give up, knowing only too well that one or more complications could compromise everything.

Stephanie's tiny body was hooked up to numerous machines around her bed. The hours dragged by. The days seemed endless. Tests were followed by more tests, examinations by more examinations. All of them were designed to determine whether the lungs were functioning more easily, whether the amount of oxygen in the blood had reached an acceptable level, whether the kidneys were affected, or whether there was any imbalance in the blood count caused by the illness or by the current treatment. The suspense was unbearable, even for the staff who were accustomed to an intensive care setting. Stephanie was hovering between life and death; she was hanging on by a thread.

This critical period lasted for ten days. The weeks that followed were also very difficult, as other complications had set in. They included a bacterial pneumonia accompanied by fluid around the lungs. This was in addition to the psychological problems caused by Stephanie having been removed from intensive care. The poor child was afraid of being alone, which was perfectly understandable considering all she had gone through. But at least her life was no longer in danger. Time helped to erase all the bad memories. Today, the only visible signs of the terrible chickenpox are a few small scars, which are normal after such an illness. Fortunately, only a few cases of this infectious illness among leukemic children are as serious as Stephanie's.

● ● ●

The period of remission enables us to discover the immeasurable reserves of strength and courage in the bodies and souls of our young patients. The parents are the first to recognize it, and it makes them very proud of their children.

"I am amazed at my daughter's strength and of that of the other young patients. They're so determined and in such control of themselves. I don't think any adult could survive what they're going through. Even their smallest gestures make us so very proud. A smile once in a while. A wink. My little girl was so sick that she hadn't smiled or laughed in a month. Then, when she saw her father make a face when he bit into a slice of lemon, she broke up laughing. She was laughing so hard she almost cried. How could I not be happy? And just a while later, how could I not be overjoyed to see Marie-Jo walking on her own after being in bed for six weeks? She was walking even though she barely had the strength. How could I not be proud when that little ten-year-old got an average of ninety-two percent after having been absent from school for five months? Just watching our child play with other normal children fills us with joy."

In order to complete the picture, I would have to relate the case history of every child who visits the outpatient clinic at Sainte-Justine Hospital. Space does not permit, which is a shame, for each in its own way is a story of heroism. They tell of trauma and despair, often illuminated by humor that is both mischievous and courageous. They have taught us better to understand the true value of life. Instead, I would like to spotlight a few examples that are engraved in the memories of all those who witnessed them.

I think of Sebastien, a five-year-old boy who was terrified of needles. To overcome his fear, he had made up a little song with the help of his mother. He would sing it every time the nurse arrived with an injection:

> When you prick me,
> I jump,
> but please don't be angry.
> When you prick me,
> I know it's to make me well,
> and that helps me to love you.

Sebastien didn't know it at the time, but from that moment on, his song would be sung by all the staff of our outpatient clinic and by the young patients who visited them.

I will also never forget Andrew, who, despite his tender age of eighteen months, was one of our veterans. One day, some journalists came to the hospital to do a report on cancer among children. It was late in the day and Andrew was the only child still at the clinic. For the benefit of the photographers, a nurse thought it might be a good idea to pretend to give him an injection, because he never cried when it was his turn. Without saying anything, she took a needle filled with an IV solution, and pretended to inject it into his hand. While all this was going on, Andrew, with his free hand, tried to take off one of his boots. When the nurse realized what he was doing, she burst out laughing. The journalists were horrified. They couldn't understand what was happening. Why was she laughing in a place like this? The nurse explained, "Andrew never gets an injection in the hand, it's always in the foot. He's only doing what he's supposed to do to prepare for the shot. In his own way, he is proving exactly what we've been telling you. These children really are exceptional."

One last anecdote. Kevin, a five-year-old with a lymphoma was playing in the waiting room with other children who, like him, had lost all their hair during treatment. He asked one of them, "You also have the concert?" Kevin had confused the word *cancer* with *concert*. His mother had to smile, realizing that there was some truth in Kevin's choice of words. For what a beautiful concert these children give with their laughter and their games.

nine

THE OUTCOME

There was a party in the hematology department; Genevieve was going home for good. She was one of the fortunate ones who had won her battle against cancer. Her doctor had waited a while before telling her the good news, but the statistics had convinced him. For Genevieve, the nightmare of treatment was over. After two years of continuous treatment, the renal tumor had finally been elminated.

That same day, we also had a brief visit from Nathalie, who was only four when we first diagnosed her illness. She is now an adolescent and she had not been to see us for several years. Her parents are still incredulous:

"We just can't believe it's true, doctor. Is there any risk of after-effects later on as a result of the treatment she has received?"

"We'll have to wait a few years before we know whether there will be any negative effects from the chemotherapy. One problem among girls is sterility; it happens in about one case in every four or five. Leukemic girls who have undergone treatment may also experience some disturbance in their menstrual cycle. As for the rest, girls who have had leukemia will be just like any other women as far as their secondary sexual characteristics are concerned; their breasts develop normally, for example. They can lead a normal sexual life."

"But what if she has children?"

"I hope she does. And you needn't worry that her children will be leukemic or abnormal as a result of her illness. A study done on over a hundred young pregnant women who had been treated for cancer when they were younger, failed to show any problems during pregnancy, any miscarriages, any detectable deformation in the children, or any other form of chronic illness. Had your child been a boy, I wouldn't have been able to tell you much because the results aren't in yet in this regard. There may be a risk of sterility, but it remains to be proven."

"Doctor, does this mean that our Nathalie is protected from ever getting cancer again?"

"No one is ever really protected from cancer, not even someone who has already had it. People who have suffered from cancer can contract it again at some point down the line. A study done on four hundred and ten patients, which was published in 1975, mentioned twenty-eight cases where a second tumor had appeared between six and twenty-one years after treatment for infantile cancer. Fifteen of these cases involved a malignant tumor. It's important to note that all of these second cancers appeared in areas that had been subjected to radiotherapy. They can, therefore, be considered as side effects of the radiotherapy. Your daughter has undergone cranial therapy and she therefore runs a small risk of contracting another tumor. There are other forms of cancer, such as Hodgkin's disease (in patients who have been treated with a combination of chemotherapy and radiotherapy) that have a tendency to reappear ten to fifteen years later in the form of acute leukemia. In general terms, the incidence of a second cancer among children is between eight and twelve percent during the two decades following treatment. This compares to an incidence of about one percent for the general population in the corresponding age category. These statistics can obviously be very disturbing, but we must face facts. In order to combat Nathalie's leukemia, we had to resort to the weapons at hand. What's more, if we consider the nature of her illness and the specific treatments she received, the risk of her contracting another cancer is small."

"All the same, doctor, it's very worrying. Will she always have to live in fear?"

"No. She has every reason to be as optimistic about the future as the next person."

"Is it possible that she'll have psychological problems as a result of her illness? Does it mean that our child will be more susceptible to mental illness?"

"No. Children who have beaten cancer adjust very quickly to a normal life. A study carried out on a hundred and forty-two people, aged over eighteen, who had similar experiences to your little girl's, showed that the majority of them had completed their university studies. Several had become professionals or business people. It also showed that most of them were bringing up families of their own."

Paradoxically, there was the case of a woman of twenty-five who had received treatment for leukemia for several years; she suffered a nervous breakdown when she learned that she was cured. She said that she had lost her reason for living, which had been her fight against cancer. It became necessary for her to find another challenge; to learn how to live again and how to take full advantage of a normal life. There was also the case, both touching and amusing, of a four-year-old boy who had lost his hair. His friends nicknamed him Kojak after the television detective, and he loved to play up to the role. When his hair grew back he lost this new identity and the prestige that went with it. It had become the biggest joy in his life. Suddenly he had to learn how to be himself again, just a little boy no different from any of his friends.

The majority of cured children leave the clinic without too much fuss and fanfare. For them, the victory has been won gradually and without any hoopla. Their medical visits become so infrequent that we sometimes have difficulty recognizing our former charges when they come in for their six- or twelve-month check ups. These visits enable us to check whether certain anomalies have arisen, such as a deviation of the spine or retarded growth in specific areas, attributable to our various treatments. More than that, though, these visits allow us to renew old friendships.

There are many other stories, however, that do not end quite so happily. One day, I had to tell an eighteen-year-old, a former diving champion, that because of the advanced state of her illness, we were going to have to amputate her left leg and part of her pelvis. For the past year she had been receiving treatment for a bone tumor. She had suffered from terrible pains in her hip, her left leg did not respond anymore, and her loss of weight and general weakness had become critical. I was afraid of how she would take this terrible news. Imagine my surprise when she accepted it without flinching. She told me she had already arrived at the same conclusion. I was expecting a crisis, and instead I found that my young patient was comforting me: "Don't worry about it. I'll get over it."

We set a date for the operation, but meanwhile an unpleasant surprise awaited us. A few days before she was to go into surgery, we found a lung metastasis that would also have to be operated on. We began with a hemipelvectomy, amputating the left leg, and then proceeded to open the chest to get at the tumor in the lung. After all that, our patient "got over it" just as she had promised. During the post-op period, she experienced phantom leg pains that she learned to master in a remarkable way: through self-hypnosis. Today, she has taken up all her old activities. She still swims and dives. She even teaches young children how to swim. These children adore her. Even more incredibly, this girl has become an exceptional skier and the envy of some of her ski-instructor friends. She has every right to be proud.

• • •

Benjamin was only a baby when he first came to us. At the age of one, he had to have an eye removed because of a malignant tumor, a retinoblastoma. All went well for a time and everyone wanted to believe that he was really cured. When he turned twelve, however, Ben began to complain of pains in his right leg. We noticed a lump, and a further examination revealed an osteosarcoma. Unhappily, this was not too unusual. Some patients who have had a retinoblastoma may be prisdisposed to another form of cancer several years after they have been cured of the first tumor. It was necessary to operate on this boy a second time. We had to amputate the leg and begin chemotherapy. Ben is cured now. He has beaten two cancers and has succeeded in overcoming two handicaps. It seems nothing can get him down. He is full of vitality, and his favourite sport is cycling. During a cyclothon in which some one thousand cyclists participated, he was among the first to finish, followed closely by his friend Daniel, who had also lost a leg to an osteosarcoma. If Ben ever participates in the Marathon of Hope, inspired by the late Terry Fox, it will be in his own way: on a bicycle rather than on foot.

When David went up against the giant Goliath, the young biblical hero didn't seem to have much of a chance of coming out of it alive. Yet armed with only a simple sling and his courage, he emerged victorious. Children who succeed in beating cancer are the little Davids of our Generation. Just a few decades ago, the young cancer victim needed extraordinary luck to beat the enemy. In the majority of cases the battle was lost.

Today our Davids are better armed to the extent that statistics give them one chance in two of beating the aggressor. Still, it is difficult if not impossible to understand how much courage it takes for them to get through it. It's hard to pick out these small warriors in a crowd of other children, despite the marks they sometimes carry from their long and difficult fight.

• • •

One chance in two. Unfortunately, that also means that half the childhood cancer victims succumb. Because a remission is now the rule rather than the exception, it is the relapse, more often than not, that heralds the threat of death. A relapse can happen at any time, without warning, in the most brutal and unexpected manner.

Lisa was pale and not at all her usual self. She was pensive. For the past two years, this fourteen-year-old had been attending the clinic for treatment for acute leukemia. She was usually bright and cheerful. Lisa often put up some resistance to the treatment, but she always came round to accepting it. As she lived quite a distance away from the city, she was under the care of a doctor in her home town who kept in touch with us.

Lisa had followed the evolution of her illness very closely. She was familiar with its coordinates, and she wanted to make all her own decisions. One day, she had made the trip to our clinic in town alone. She was afraid her blood count had reached a dangerous level. Having had the same problem the year before, she wanted to believe that it was only an anomaly caused by some medicinal toxicity. Upon examining her, I noticed that she was very pale and that her spleen was palpable. There was no choice; we had to examine the bone marrow to determine the exact nature of the problem. The results were conclusive: Lisa had suffered a relapse. How could I explain to this young girl that she would not be able to return to the country; that she had to remain in the hospital? She could sense my discomfort immediately, but I had no choice, I had to tell her the truth.

"Lisa, the blood count shows that—"
"You don't have to tell me. I've had a relapse, haven't I?"

A tear fell on her cheek. She said nothing more, but listened calmly while I explained that we would have to start treating her again with different drugs and that she would have to remain with us for a few days. The nausea would return and, once again, she would lose her hair. There was hardly any reaction. Lisa seemed crushed, and understandably so. After talking for about thirty minutes, she prepared to leave the outpatient clinic. With one foot out the door, her head lowered, she said in a choked voice, "Anyway, I know what it all means." I asked her to come back and explain.

"Doctor, I know . . ."
"You know what?"
"I know that I'm going to die."

She then started sobbing and threw herself in my arms. I felt the pain that was tearing her apart. I felt so helpless. I offered her a chair and sat down myself. I asked her too look me in the eye.

"It's true that you're running a greater risk of dying now that you've had a relapse. But never accept that it's over. Lisa, you're going to have to be very strong. We're going to have to start building and fighting all over again."

She understood that there really was no other choice. For my part, I had to find a solution. It was then that I thought of trying a bone-marrow transplant. This form of treatment wasn't available locally at that time, but I felt that Lisa could profit from it. I had to speak to her parents and her brothers and sisters immediately to bring them up to date and to begin preliminary studies. As soon as Lisa had a remission (when the chances for success would be greater), we would go ahead with the marrow transplant. Fate decided otherwise. Lisa died from an infectious complication in August, 1980, some three months after the relapse, without ever having been granted a remission.

● ● ●

Daniel, aged fourteen, had undergone surgery three months earlier to remove an abdominal lymphoma. The surgeon believed he had succeeded in removing everything, and subsequent examinations did not reveal any spreading of the tumor. Still Daniel complained of various pains, which could have been side effects from the chemotherapy and radiotherapy he'd been subjected to recently. But Daniel feared the worst. He was afraid that his tumor was coming back and that he'd have to be operated on again. Yet another examination confirmed his fears; the tumor had indeed returned. It could be felt when examining his stomach, which was already so badly bruised. There was more: his blood also contained malignant cells. Were his splitting headaches the result of these cells infiltrating his brain? The illness had spread, becoming more generalized. How would he take the news?

"Daniel, I don't want to lie to you. It seems that the tumor we removed is trying to come back."
"No! It's not possible."

These were the only words he spoke. Sitting in his chair, he stared at the floor as if not wanting to hear the discouraging words that I was forced to speak. His mother, who was by his side, took his hand, trying to comfort him while she attempted to control her own emotions.

"Daniel," I continued, "we have to change the treatment, but we won't operate. I can't promise that we'll never have to operate, but we won't for now. We will, however, have to change your chemotherapy by switching to something more radical."

The boy listened, but his mind was elsewhere. While he understood what was being said to him, he didn't believe that all would go as well as his doctor wanted him to think it would. A few tears trickled down his cheeks. He remained absolutely still, his eyes riveted on the same spot. After a long silence, he spoke:

"What happens if this treatment doesn't work like you think it will?"

"Well, we'll have to try some new treatments, like the ones we administer in super doses. But we won't start with those. We'll start with a more simple form of treatment in the hope that that will do the trick."

Daniel seemed to accept what he was being told, but still he didn't move. The only sound was his breathing. Suddenly, his mother who had bravely kept herself in check until then, burst out crying. She threw her arms around him and buried her head in his shoulder. The roles were reversed; she was now seeking comfort from her child. Daniel agreed to undergo treatment. As the days passed, it was impossible to escape the fact that his illness was getting worse. Two weeks later, it was all over. The lymphoma had spread and Daniel breathed his last.

It is often easier to accept the initial confirmation of the illness than it is to accept a relapse. In many cases it is then that all hope seems to vanish. The relapse means that the patient will have to receive more injections and experience more suffering. It means that the hair will fall out again, with its inevitable effect on the child's self-image. For some, it means surgery. Above all, it means that the invisible enemy is still present, determined to win the battle. It means that, once again, the patients must face the unknown, the unpredictable. It means they have to try all over again, and they sometimes ask themselves whether it's really all worth it.

The bad news of a relapse opens wounds that have barely healed. The courage of the victim and the parents is once again put to the test. Are they going to give up or can they find the strength to fight again?

Over the next few weeks they will have to draw upon hidden reserves of strength. The parents no longer have any illusions about their child's capacity to resist, or about the resources of medicine. Statements such as "our child is very strong" or "science is so advanced today" no longer have any meaning for them. They live with a harsh reality staring them in the face. Despite these setbacks, however, they must continue to fight, rising to every occasion. The battle is not over yet. Surely there is some glimmer of hope.

Should death occur after the relapse, the period between these two events can be quite prolonged. It can last several months or several years. During this phase, not only the child, but also the parents may have an extremely rough time of it. They will have to learn to accept a series of events that can very easily make them lose faith. There are the possibilities of sudden deterioration and unforeseen developments. During the period of relapse, parents and children must learn to take both the good news and the bad news without ever losing hope.

• • •

In August of 1979, Isabelle was in remission; the bone-marrow test had confirmed it. The staff in the hematology department was ecstatic. What made it all the more extraordinary was that this was the third remission for this leukemic patient, who was only five years old. The success was also due to a new drug, 5-AZA-2'-deoxycytidine. What fantastic news! We had been working on this drug for several months, and the result of our efforts was the crowning glory of six years of research. The researchers on our team had been working all-out on biochemical studies and animal tests in order to perfect the drug. Now, here was our first success in a human being. One of our interns, who had worked closely with Isabelle during every stage of her treatment, had the pleasure of telling the child and her parents the good news. They were thrilled. Isabelle in remission! A new victory. Yet we all knew that we had only won a battle, not the war. We had to maintain that remission, this time for good. Knowing this did not detract from our joy or our hopes of having discovered an extraordinary weapon for keeping leukemic cells in check. This success was going to permit us to learn the true effectiveness of the new drug, and help us to determine its use in stubborn cases of leukemia, either by itself or in combination with other drugs.

A short time later, however, Isabelle suffered yet another relapse. It was a terrible blow, both for the child—for whom the remission had meant the possibility of ending treatment—and for her parents, who had so desperately wanted to believe in miracles. It almost goes without saying that the medical team would also dearly have loved to believe that their professional success was something irrefutable and definite.

THE LUMBAR PUNCTURE

The multiple complications associated with a relapse oblige us to resort to drastic treatments and to techniques that are, to some extent, disagreeable to and even painful for the young patient. One such treatment is the spinal tap or lumbar puncture, which remains an essential step in easing the chronic headaches caused by leukemic cells invading the brain. The lumbar puncture enables us to withdraw some spinal fluid, which is examined for leukemic cells. Medication that is introduced into the spinal canal at the same time destroys any malignant cells lodged in the meninges. It also alleviates the headaches. Unfortunately, this meningitis has a tendency to return, necessitating more spinal taps. For this reason, some leukemic children undergo dozens of lumbar punctures. In the case of Julie, who died at the age of ten, the total was 120. We will never forget this little child who, before each episode of leukemic meningitis, would say to her parents, "Mommy, Daddy, I hear a big wind blowing in my head." In Julie's case we had no alternatives. Had we not resorted to the spinal tap, the pain would have been intolerable and the other symptoms much greater.

What is a lumbar puncture? Is it a simple treatment like so many of the others? Here is the view of one mother:

"A lumbar puncture for a leukemic child is a method of treatment that consists of freezing an area at the base of the spine in order to insert a long needle into the spinal canal. The needle withdraws a white liquid for analysis, and medicine is inserted. In some cases it only takes five minutes. In others it seems like an eternity. Does the child suffer? Yes, but not terribly. When the doctor freezes the area, there is a slight prick. When he inserts the needle there is a little pressure. But still it's not as simple as all that. The children must remain absolutely still; they mustn't move at all, sometimes for hours on end. They cry, they complain, and even scream for long periods at a time. It takes all their energy, strength and resistance, because they're afraid. Children often develop a phobia about the lumbar puncture because they can't see what's happening behind their backs. For these children, it's not just a question of pain, it's one of not being able to see what's going on.

"For other children, however, a spinal tap is nothing special, nothing terribly dramatic. They don't even need their parents there. Whenever their presence is required, it's usually the mother who's there. She can't show any nervousness, she can't faint when she sees the needle going into her child's body. No. A mother must encourage and support her child. She needs to be reassuring. After undergoing this supreme test, she may learn, at times only days later, that she has to go through it all again. It's not just us, the mothers and the kids, who hate spinal taps. I've got to include the doctors. A lumbar puncture demands supreme concentration on their part. They have to work meticulously and slowly, always guarding against the slightest movement on the part of the child. [The child's back must be rounded so that the needle can enter easily; if the child moves, or straightens his back, the needle may be blocked, thus hindering the procedure.] The doctors must have been through this many times before. How else could they remain unmoved by the cries of their young patients. How else can they overcome the stress that this delicate operation invariably produces in all concerned?"

• • •

The period following a relapse is riddled with problems. I often think of them as ambushes. The physical resistance of the child is weakened and, as a result, he is more susceptible to infectious complications. Today it is pneumonia. A few weeks later a mysterious infection may induce a high fever, which has to be treated with antibiotics. Perhaps tomorrow there will be a nasal hemorrhage, which means an emergency dash to the hospital for a transfusion of healthy platelets. The child's blood count, which tends to fluctuate during this period, has to be watched constantly. All of these factors result in numerous visits to the outpatient clinic, a longer stay in the hospital, starting annoying examinations all over again, repeated marrow punctures, and a new series of injections. And all this time, fear sets in. Fear of needles, even if you know that it is not going to hurt, fear of new complications, fear of missing school and, probably, fear of dying.

"I don't want to die," pleaded Kanoukone, an eighteen-year-old leukemic girl who had suffered a relapse. She was also the victim of an infectious complication that had sent her into a state of shock. Her blood pressure was at zero. She remained conscious, however, and worried. Several doctors and nurses were around her bed. "Hold on, Kanoukone. You'll feel better in a few minutes," they urged.

Meanwhile, a nurse administered an IV solution, which was not easy because Kanoukone's veins had all but disappeared. She needed blood quickly.

"But doctor, we haven't completed the analysis yet."
"It doesn't matter. Just make sure it's the same blood type and bring it to me. Do it right now."

Would the blood that we were going to inject into her veins give Kanoukone the strength she needed? The hospital room was suddenly transformed into an intensive care unit. There were all kinds of people, and equipment of every description filling it. Kanoukone's blood pressure was still zero.

Eventually, Kanoukone started to feel better. All of our efforts had paid off. But what did she really have? Was it a serious infection that had reduced her to this state or was it an internal hemorrhage? Even so, luck was on our side for, little by little, she was improving.

During the long hours of intensive care, Kanoukone kept repeating, over and over, "I don't want to die. I don't want to die." The only family she had were her two brothers. They gave her moral support while trying to hide their own tears. One held onto her hand, the other her foot. Kanoukone remained hooked up to numerous serums, which took over where the blood left off. For the moment, they were her only hope.

● ● ●

A father once told me, after a lung complication had suddenly threatened his son's life:

"There are difficult periods that force us to live one day at a time. But what really upsets me are the things that force us to live minute-by-minute, never knowing what's in store for us at the next turn, or whether our son will stop breathing from one second to the next. It's something that I have to overcome. But it's very hard to take."

Other people refuse to face up to reality, such as the mother who only wanted to look at her son, to forget the illness that had ravaged him:

"I don't want to know anything about tomorrow or the day after. I no longer think that he's going to die. I look at him today, and that's enough."

Among the parents who do worry about the next day, there is a common preoccupation: will their child see another Christmas? This holiday has become a sacred objective that they must attain. They refuse to think of celebrating such an important day without their child. One mother told me:

"Josie is really an exceptional little girl. One day, she met Santa Claus and he tried to find out what she really wanted for Christmas. A game? No. A doll? No. A pair of skates? No. She wanted her health, lots of health. I tell you, Santa didn't know how to answer her. He probably would have loved to have been able to grant her wish. Josie knew that she was asking a lot from Santa. She knew that she wasn't like the other children, that she was ill.

"But she had to see Christmas. And Santa Claus, with the blessing of little Jesus, must grant her the most beautiful present of all—her health. Christmas, however, doesn't always bring miracles."

● ● ●

In the shadows that border death, there is another event that has to be taken into consideration: that of the metamorphosis, the physical and emotional changes that occur in the children. It takes many forms, and all patients who enter the long and painful terminal stage are subject to it. The physical changes are not simply a question of hair loss, but may involve a pronounced cachexia, a deformity brought about by the size of a tumoral mass, a disfiguration linked to an uncontrollable infection, or a shocking paleness. There can be emotional changes as well, such as a psychological regression where the child begins to behave like a baby again.

There comes a moment when even the parents feel like strangers with their child. One day, a mother who had just lost her child confided in me:

"You told us a lot of things, doctor, when you were treating our daughter, but you never really dwelt on the change that occurs in these children. As time went by our daughter became unrecognizable. She was no longer the girl we had known, the one who was always playing and laughing, and who loved to go to school. No. Towards the end, she was not our little girl. Her eyes were so sad and empty, her face was lifeless. She had regressed so much, and her little body had shrunk. At the same time, the tumor got so big towards the end that my husband and I had the impression that all we could see was this terrible monstrosity. No, our baby didn't die last week. She died over a month ago. During the last few weeks we were in the presence of a strange extension of our daughter."

As I mentioned earlier, the metamorphosis takes different forms. Fortunately, in the majority of cases the changes are bearable. They are rarely truly hideous, such as is the case when the eyes bulge from their sockets or when the mouth is so deformed that the saliva trickles un-controllably down the chin, or when the tumoral mass is so large it dwarfs the body. Cancer shows no mercy and it does not always allow a person to die with dignity.

I must repeat that these extreme transformations are the exception rather than the rule. In the majority of cases, there is merely a gradual transformation brought about by excessive weight loss. Parents are only human and, in some of the worst cases, they may be so traumatized by the profound physical changes that they have diffculty in relating to their son or daughter. They prefer to remember their child as he or she looked when in good health, with big eyes open wide on a world that was waiting to be conquered. The parents must face up to these changes because this child, even though transformed, is the same child they have always known, with the same needs for love and security. They must leap the barriers, tear down the screens, and love their children even more, giving all the tenderness they have to give. In doing so, they will themselves experience a metamorphosis. For their children, they will become the expression of love itself.

● ● ●

The pain will become particularly pronounced during the terminal phase. More than a quarter of cancer victims will experience it to a great degree. Half of them will experience it to some degree. Only one in four will be spared. The pain takes various forms: it can press against the cushioning of the bones, which feels like an abcess ready to burst. It can pinch a nerve membrane, which feels like being squeezed by pincers. It can feel like the brain is swelling in the narrow confines of the skull.

The pain can be so intense that even those around the patient seem to feel it, as though they also had a headache, or a pain in their bones or their stomach. They wish they could take on the burden of pain instead of the child. They are sometimes tempted to put an end to the nightmare. One day, a distraught father who had watched his child suf-fer terribly came to me and pleaded, "Doctor, if you don't put an end to it, I will. We wouldn't let a dog suffer like that. Why do you persist?" He choked up, sobbing. He suddenly realized that he was wishing his son dead. The realization was too much for him. Had he become a cruel, unnatural father? No. He loved his son so much that he wanted to spare him; he preferred to see him die than to continue suffering so. You must not believe that the pain is always so severe. It comes and it goes. It plays on the nerves. One day it's intolerable, then it disappears, only to reappear later. It can also move around the body. Today, it's in the right leg. Tomorrow it may be in the left leg, the stomach, or the head.

Not all cancerous children suffer to the same degree. When the pain becomes excessive, we take major steps to suppress it. We, the doctors, believe it is necessary to combat the pain with every means at our disposal. That's our first duty at this stage. Cancerous children must not be left to suffer.

What can we really do for the pain? Even living a normal life obliges us to accept a certain amount of pain—ask anyone suffering from arthritis. We also experience sharp pains once in a while, when we twist an ankle, for example. We're all familiar with pain. However, it can become acute to the point where it's intolerable, and that's when modern medicine must intervene. We have to resort to drugs, starting with minor analgesics and moving up to major ones, if necessary. With cancer patients the pain can be so intense and tenacious that it very quickly demands powerful palliatives. Simple aspirin are not enough, neither is codeine. One has to use morphine, which is taken orally (a Brompton cocktail) or intravenously, drop by drop.

This last method is almost always effective. It permits us to control the pain to a satisfactory degree. If the pain returns, we increase the dosage until it is clear that the child is no longer suffering. This worries some parents, who ask us whether their child will become a morphine addict. The risk of this is really a theoretical one. In all the years that I've been a doctor, I've neither seen nor heard of a cancerous child of any age who has become dependent on morphine, much less an addict. As soon as the pain disappears, it's possible for us to cut the morphine without provoking any withdrawal symptoms. No longer suffering, the child asks for nothing more and is usually happy to get on with living.

It's not always the same with adults. With them, there are often many side effects from morphine, ranging from discomfort to dependancy. Be this as it may, morphine remains the most powerful analgesic for both adults and children. It is more effective than hydromorphine, oxymorphine, nalpubine, and even heroin.

Our method of administering morphine has changed somewhat with time. Today, we give it on a regular basis, that is to say, we introduce it into the blood at a constant level and in sufficient strength to kill the pain. The daily dose of morphine can become quite impressive, for we only cut it off when it's evident the patient is no longer suffering. Some young children who are going through the terminal phase become partially resistant to morphine after several weeks or months of taking the drug.

These children might receive a daily dose of morphine that is ten to fifty times stronger than that we would give an adult suffering from coronary thrombosis. With such a dose, it is possible to ease the pain without provoking too many undesirable side effects. We now have access to clinics that specialize in the phenomenon of pain and to experimental techniques ranging from pharmacological methods, such as the use of endorphine, to the most advanced psychological methods.

For some time now, self-hypnosis has played an important role in combatting pain. Everyone knows that anxiety accentuates pain and that thinking about something else can make the situation more bearable. Pain is a sensation, a real sensation that corresponds to precise causes and, as such, can be mastered. Whenever chemical substances prove to be ineffective, whenever surgery plays only a palliative role in interrupting pain, it is worth fully exploiting one's innermost resources. Motivation can become such a positive element that it enables one to support an even higher level of pain.

Hypnosis operates by neuropsychic mechanisms and can be extraordinarily effective in the treatment of pain. This form of therapy becomes even more interesting when one considers that it can be practised by the patient, even if the patient is a child. We have known children, aged five to ten, who have been able to resort to self-hypnosis and who have succeeded in reducing the pain and worry brought about by examinations and injections. Older children can learn to reduce the phantom pains that follow an amputation to the point where they have no further need of analgesics. Self-hypnosis is also used to control nausea and vomiting following chemotherapy.

Several other methods of mastering or combatting pain are also being tried among cancerous adults, but these cannot be used for children. I refer to the use of marijuana, more complex methods of relaxation, biofeedback, acupuncture, and electrotherapy. None of these are easy to apply to young patients. We must concentrate, therefore, on methods that can be applied to children if we are to relieve their suffering. Thus the two most important methods are still the use of chemical substances, such as morphine, and self-hypnosis.

If we allow ourselves to believe that we can overcome physical pain, can we say the same of psychological suffering? How can we give back a leg to a young boy who had dreams of becoming a hockey star? How can we restore the sight of a small girl who is blind because we had to remove a tumor that was threatening her life? How can we tell a child that he will soon feel better because of the drugs that we're giving him when, all in all, he would rather be out playing with his friends?

Is it possible to ease the suffering of mothers and fathers who have to stand by helplessly as death claims their children? They have spent months, perhaps years, living in hope. Now there is no hope left. There is only the waiting. Waiting for the doctor to come by to tell them how it's going. Waiting for the day to end. Waiting for the next day to begin. Waiting to see what that day will bring. Waiting, all the while knowing that death is imminent.

As death draws nearer, the parents, more often than not, adopt an attitude of disbelief. It seems inconceivable to them that their child is going to be cut down before reaching maturity. Once they've accepted it, or at least recognized it, fear takes over. They're afraid on behalf of their child, and they project to the child their own fear of death. The uncertainty over exactly how their child is going to die also frightens them.

As for the children, they accept death much more serenely. They do not have the same perception of death as adults do. They are not old enough for death to have taken on the metaphysical dimensions that make it so terrible to adults. That's not to say they're unaware of what is happening. We're always torn apart when we hear children say things like, "Now I will never be a child like the others," or "I don't think I'll ever get any older," or "What will you do with my toys when I'm gone?"

The end can come quite quietly, providing the pain can be kept in check. On realizing that they are entering the terminal phase, some children refuse treatment, even though they know what this means for them. Some speak quite openly of death and, in their own way, draw up their wills: "Daddy, you will take good care of my dog, Chico, when I'm gone, won't you?" Some pass away without saying a word, without any warning at all, while their parents are asleep in a chair, or when there is absolutely no one in the room. It's almost as if they planned it that way. Still others will cling to life only until their parents return to the room.

• • •

Alan's parents were praying as they had never prayed before. Their leukemic son, a teenager, was coming to the end of his long illness; he had fallen into a semi-coma. It was calm in the hospital room; day and night no longer existed. They were living in a time zone completely removed from that of the outside world. The minutes ticked away. The heavy silence was broken only by Alan's hoarse breathing and the steady throbbing of a pump administering morphine.

His parents took turns holding their son's hand, to show that they were there supporting him, that they were with him, that they loved him. After several hours in this unusual state of symbiosis—it seemed like several days—the father looked at his son for a long time. He moved closer and put his head close to Alan's, whispering in his ear: "Let go, son. Yes, you can do it now. You've fought long enough."

Alan seemed to be in a deep sleep, but he opened his eyes and looked at his grieving parents. In a voice that was barely audible, he whispered, "Daddy, Mommy, thank you. Thank you for everything." These were his last words. He fell asleep, lost consciousness, and died the next morning. He had finally let go and he died with the grace that had characterized his life.

The death of some children causes hospital workers to witness scenes that are particularly heartbreaking. I will never forget the circumstances surrounding the death of Andrea, a little girl of four. It came at a time when I was just starting out in oncology—the speciality of cancer. Andrea had been suffering for eighteen months from a cruel tumor, a neuroblastoma.

She had never been able to get the upper hand on the cancer that was wasting her body. Her parents seemed unable to accept the inevitable outcome of the illness. Nevertheless, deep down they knew that the end would come one day. Over a period of a few days, Andrea's condition became desperate. Her body was completely wracked by the tumor. Early one morning, after having slept at the hospital, the father returned to his child's room to be told that Andrea's breathing had become much worse during the night. I had been called to the child's bed. I could see that her condition was deteriorating by the minute. Her breathing had become so bad that to ponder any improvement at all was just wishful thinking.

The father stood by, helplessly watching. He had suffered terribly in the past year, losing his father, his brother, and two young nephews as the result of accidents. This latest blow was too much for him. Suddenly, he grabbed me by the arm and shouted, "Doctor, do something. Make her breathe!" Only God could grant his wish. Andrea died a few minutes later. Her mother arrived seconds too late. She threw herself on the lifeless body of her only child, wrapped her in her arms, and cried, "No, my little girl isn't dead. She's still with me!"

While the mother wept uncontrollably, the father walked to the window and, shaking his fists at the sky, he began to swear. He swore like I have never heard anyone swear before or since. Whenever I remember this scene, even though it took place many years ago, I get shivers up my spine.

Another time, it was the day after Christmas, I had hardly arrived at home from the hospital when the phone rang. They were calling me about Kevin, a five-year-old who had been diagnosed as having a lymphoma about nine months previously. He was already in the terminal phase. Although Kevin had passed a happy Christmas with his family, that day, nothing was going well. It was only a few blocks to his house from mine, so I went over. By the time I arrived his breathing had become difficult and he was fighting desperately not to fall asleep. He refused to get into bed, preferring to sit in an armchair that dwarfed him.

Kevin's eyes were heavy and bloodshot. The results of the latest examination were conclusive; the pneumonia had gained ground. I conferred with the parents and we agreed to follow through with a decision taken earlier. We weren't going to resort to any special techniques. We weren't going to do anything out of the ordinary. We would keep the child as comfortable as possible. The end would come here at Kevin's home, surrounded by his family, rather than at the hospital. I gave him a mini-dose of analgesics. He calmed down and stretched out on a divan. His breathing was becoming slower, lighter; at times it even stopped for a while. It looked as though the child was about to leave us. It was now impossible for us to hold on to him. His parents were kneeling on either side of the divan. Each held one of his hands and whispered over and over again, "Kevin, I love you. I love you, Kevin, . . ." Cradled in this litany of love, he departed from this world.

It's difficult to lose children such as Lisa, Daniel, Andrea, and Kevin. Sometimes when doctors see the suffering around them, they're tempted to give in to the futility of it all. The suffering at times renders them helpless. In my case, I think of Chantal, of Patrick, and of all the others who no longer need us, the ones who beat cancer. Today, they only need space, the sun, the wind and the waves, and I am content to know that not all our efforts are in vain.

To meet children every day who are only passing through this world is to enroll in a school of life. Despite all our money, science, and technical expertise, we must listen to the messages left us by these transient children. Nobody in the world can really understand the meaning of life until they have held the hand of one of these little heroes at the moment of death. No judge should pass sentence, no politican should legislate, no philosopher should pass on the fruits of his meditation until he has been with one of these children at the end of his short journey on this earth. For it would only be then that they could really appreciate the true value of life. This realization makes us respect all that life entails and all those who share this life with us.

ten

THE PSYCHOLOGY OF CANCER
by Suzanne Douesnard, Psychologist

Whenever children are suddenly attacked by leukemia or cancer, their whole world is shattered. What was once a warm, magical world full of fairytales and wonder becomes black, dark, and full of monsters, syringes, needles and masks. The masks of the doctors and the nurses, but also the masks worn by the parents to protect themselves and their children from the harsh truth. Masks that hide tears behind smiles. Good-bye innocence. Goodbye magic. Goodbye childhood.

The child must live in pain, at least for a while. The youngster will feel sadness, boredom, anger, and fear. Fear of being left alone in the hospital, of being apart from his or her parents for the first time. Fear of all these new people who seem so friendly but who are nevertheless strangers. Fear of what is being done to them.

The staff talks about things the child can't understand and doesn't even want to hear. They insist he go to bed when he wants to play. Then they wake him up when he would prefer to sleep. They weigh him, measure him, give him tests, they look at him, study him, question him, and they don't seem to listen to what he says. They prick his fingers, his bottom, his hands, his arms, his back. They make him swallow a lot of bitter pills, and they don't even crush them up in jam. They take his photograph with huge machines that don't look anything like his father's camera. What's more, his father's camera never made his hair fall out. Everything is a source of fear.

What can one say about the feelings of loneliness? The child misses her mother, who has gone home to take care of her little brother. She misses her father, who can't visit because he has to work. She misses her brother. Sure they fight sometimes, but she loves him all the same. She also misses her dog, which she loves to scratch behind the ears. Will the dog still love her when she leaves the hospital and comes home? She misses school and worries that she'll miss the whole year. Will her schoolfriends remember her?

The feeling of guilt is a very important factor in the emotional makeup of sick children. They feel guilty because they are causing problems for their parents. They feel they are to blame for the parents' sadness, their worry, their red eyes, and the lines on their faces. All the youngsters feel guilty about some of their past actions or desires. They can very easily come to believe that their illness is some kind of well-deserved punishment.

Crowning all these fears and worries is the terrible anxiety related to the sickness itself, and to death. Is the illness serious? Is it curable? When will they operate and cut me up? Will I die? All of these questions haunt the children, even though they are not always clearly expressed. The children try to push these questions to the back of their minds, but they return to torment them. As a direct result of this anxiety, children can react badly to hospitalization or treatment. They can have trouble eating or sleeping. They can misbehave or become moody. Is it any wonder that they sometimes blow up and lose their tempers, at times even violently? Is it really surprising that at other times they will cry at the drop of a hat, unable to hide their feelings?

A child's reaction to illness will vary according to age, personality, strengths, and weaknesses. It also depends on the attitudes of the parents and others around the child. Emotional reactions are translated into changes in character or behaviour, which can either be temporary or permanent. A sick child can become agitated and fretful, gregarious or withdrawn, he or she can play the fool or be extremely serious. A child can become aggressive, manipulative, and even tyrannical. Some are also demanding, egocentric, or regressive. A child can display all the normal traits of a child, or a maturity that is out of all proportion to its age. A child may complain about the treatment he is receiving or be surprisingly understanding about it. And a child may either keep its emotions under control or flare up at the least little thing.

Certain children adopt an attitude of indifference and bravado. Nothing seems to worry them and they are always bright and cheerful. This attitude is often a cover-up for panic, worry, and sadness; children also learn to wear masks. All of these reactions and emotions are demonstrated to varying degrees by every sick child. They are normal, but one must pay close attention to them and be prepared to understand them.

Will a child be marked forever by the traumatic experience of having cancer? I've lost track of how many parents have asked this question. It almost goes without saying that an experience as painful and as upsetting as cancer cannot be lived through without leaving some mark. Leukemia and cancer are not bad dreams. They are a reality. There is no doubt that whatever children experience during this stage of their lives will be integrated into the total sum of their experiences and will be part of what makes them unique human beings.

It should be stressed that this experience can, ultimately, also be a positive one. If a child and its family use it correctly, all pulling together, the experience can help enrich the lives of all concerned. Compassion, maturity, the capacity for empathizing, learning to listen to oneself and to others, living life to the fullest, recognizing and appreciating human values; all of these qualities can be developed to become an integral part of the personality of the cancerous child.

Of course, the experience can also cause a child to worry over its physical well being. Never again will he or she be able to hide behind that old saying, "It can't happen to me." It is important to remember, however, that the child's whole personality will be influenced by other experiences, not only this one. Their personalities will be the sum of all experiences, happy and sad, positive and negative, just as it is with all human beings.

Leukemic or cancerous children are still children. They express normal needs, which can be summed up in three words: *to be loved*. Just like any other child, these youngsters have a deep understanding of life and a remarkable capacity to adapt. They have their own particular needs, difficulties, problems, and little quirks, but they are first and foremost children.

Now that we've defined who the sick child is, let's look at one particular dimension of the young cancer patient—the physical image the child has of himself or herself. For it is a body that has suddenly become sick that is at the centre of their human experience. What happens when that body is subjected to numerous tests and observations? When it is altered by massive doses of medicine? When it is assaulted and sometimes even mutilated by surgery? What effect does this have on that physical image, and how does it affect the personality of the child?

That a person's physical image is linked to the body is considered to be a global psychological experience. The body is the base and the centre of all emotions, and of the organization of relations with others. From the earliest age, a child must come to grips with the complex and difficult task of developing its bodily image. This involves organizing both the inner self and relationships with others.

The infant is first of all conscious of bodily sensations, both pleasant and unpleasant, such as hunger, satiety, heat, cold, and so on. This is followed by an awareness of the different parts of the body in terms of function and movement, so that it can integrate them into the definite entity that is its body. The child discovers its thumb and mouth, the movement of its hands, the sound of its voice, and so on. At the same time, as a result of the relationship with its mother or other nurturing figure, it gradually learns that it is a distinct person, and the child begins to act or react accordingly.

This development is of extreme importance because it is at the base of the emotional organization of the individual. It plants the idea that the individual must learn to take care of himself or herself, to function in the world, and enter into relationships with other people.

Thus when children become ill, it is not only their bodies that are affected, but their whole beings, at every level. Their emotions, their relationships with others, their self-images, and how they perceive the world, are all unbalanced. Even before it is defined, the illness confuses messages the children receive from their bodies. They're tired, their legs give way, they hurt. How are they to interpret these strange new signals? Their opinions of themselves may already be weakened, and the ways they have of dealing with others may change. For example, they may be frightened of giving the impression that they are "soft" because they can't run as quickly as the other children. They don't like themselves. They are afraid of being rejected by their friends, and may therefore withdraw from the group to amuse themselves in solitude. Or, as a result of the pain, they may get sulky and aggressive, becoming impossible to play with. Their parents lose patience with them, and the children then fear they are unloved.

The child's body, which has become a stranger to him, is now the focal point of his whole world. His parents, as only parents can, watch him closely for the slightest change, the smallest sign. They worry about everything. Has he got a fever? Do his legs hurt? Never before have they watched him so closely. They touch him, examine him, but what can he tell the people who are watching over him?

Medical people are also taking a lot of interest in his body. But, unlike his parents, they are not content merely to observe and analyze him. They hurt him! How can a child possibly understand—a child so naturally fearful of pain—that it's often necessary to suffer in order to get well? They hurt him because they love him. Is this the logic of adults?

The body, which has become the source of suffering and the centre of attention, undergoes changes. It becomes different, indeed, even unrecognizable. It is thinner, paler, more lined and bruised. The hair falls out, and sometimes the body is even mutilated by surgery. It all has an impact on the image the young patient has of himself. The strangeness and the new look of his body temporarily threatens his equilibrium, provoking hostility and anxiety. The child no longer has any reference points in his attitude towards himself or others.

The child must change the image he had of himself when his body was well to the reality of what it has become. If he can succeed in this, he will have a realistic concept of himself and he will be able to maintain, or rediscover his self-esteem. He will still be sad and angry, but he won't always be in a state of acute anxiety. He will also be able to re-establish satisfactory relationships with those around him. If he does not succeed in recognizing and accepting the changes in his body, he can easily become frustrated, depressed, and anxious.

One thing is certain, it will all depend on his intellectual and emotional resources and the reactions of those around him; people whom he loves, people who are important in his eyes. The child is afraid of being rejected, of not being loved any more. These fears give rise to an anxiety that is much more important than that caused by the illness itself. Of course, it is often very difficult for the parents not to react strongly when their child's arms and legs become so thin. Or when they see his little bare head. These only serve to remind them that their child is terribly ill. The child is always on the look-out for these reactions and he often misinterprets them. He easily feels rejected. It is essential, therefore, that the child is made to understand that his parents' love is in no way linked to whether he has hair or rosy cheeks, or is in good physical shape.

He must feel accepted for what he is, without hair, and with all his sadness and anger. He must know that his parents understand him, that he has the right to be sad and angry, and that he has the right to show it.

Perhaps now is the time to discuss the temporary loss of hair. Modern medicine offers a chance of life for the leukemic or cancerous child, but the loss of hair is part of the price that has to be paid. Everyone, even the children, accept this as a fair price. All the same, the doctors, their assistants, and the parents should be aware of the demands that it puts on the young patient. Because the hair grows back, and because the loss does not entail physical pain, one tends to neglect the psychological impact of this temporary baldness.

The image one projects is of extreme importance in our society. We go to a lot of trouble to modify our appearances and make our bodies conform to the ideals of our society, or even to set them apart. For example, our style of dress, makeup, hairstyle and hair colour, are all devices we use to project the image we wish to show the world. This image can define lifestyle, financial status, cultural standing, and values. We are often judged by other people according to this image. As a result of personality, values, and environment, we choose to present one image as opposed to another. The images we project can, therefore, vary according to our circumstances. Moreover, according to personality, a person may choose to accentuate one part of his or her body over another. The hair is often used to change the image we wish to project in that it reflects our personalities. It can be long, short, straight, curly, blond, brown, and so on. It can frame the face or hide it. It can make one look serious or frivolous. It can make one look older or younger.

A child is no different in this regard. Hair is very important and he uses it to project what he is, what he would like to be, and how he would like to appear to others. The loss of his hair, therefore, can give rise to an important psychological crisis that can have profound repercussions for the personal life of the child, as well as for his relationships with others. Psychologically, he feels naked, as naked as his bald head.

The severity of the crisis varies according to age; it is most severe among adolescents. It would be wrong to believe, however, that the small child remains indifferent to this transformation. Among very young children, under three years of age, the loss of hair can even complicate the normal development of body image. Among young children of school age, the crisis can be overcome relatively quickly, providing the child remains convinced of his parent's love and he is accepted by his schoolfriends. It therefore becomes very important that the young patient be reintegrated as soon as possible into both his school environment and his usual social circle. Some parents tend to keep their children at home to protect them from the stares and unkind remarks of other children. The sick child can interpret this attitude as a rejection on his parents' part, as though they refuse to accept the way he now looks. He feels that they are keeping him away from others because he has become ugly, because they are ashamed of him. In his mind, this also confirms that he has really been rejected by the others, which is not necessarily the case.

As a result of this feeling of rejection, sadness and depression set in. Behavioural problems may arise. Wouldn't it be better to prepare the child for a return to school and give him all the encouragement you can? It's always possible to inform the other children in advance so that they can give him a warm welcome. If there are any negative comments or reactions, you can always console him. You must give him the support to help him grow from his experience.

It is so important to understand what leukemic or cancerous children are going through and how it affects their behaviour and emotions. Our knowledge should permit us to help and love them all the more.

eleven

A NEW BEGINNING

To lose a child must be the most painful thing in life to overcome. It's as if one has to watch helplessly while part of oneself is savagely destroyed. We cannot lose an extension of ourselves without feeling profound grief. This grief is difficult to measure and is in no way proportionate to the age of the deceased. You might think it's more painful to lose an older child than it is to lose a baby or an infant, but when we see parents at the time of their loss, this kind of arithmetic just doesn't add up.

The great majority of parents whose children are carried off by cancer come to know a difficult period and some realize that they now have a new battle to fight. This time the enemy is no longer the illness, but the hurt that takes a different form every day.

The parents will be sorely tried in the months and perhaps years to come. In the following paragraphs, I will try to describe the five stages that I see the majority of parents going through following the death of a child: the great feeling of emptiness; then, 2) anger; 3) depression; 4) loneliness; and finally, 5) a return to a more normal life.

Immediately after the death of a child, whom they have taken care of and watched over for so long, the first emotion felt by parents is one of great emptiness. The feelings of parents who have lost a child are also tragic. They forget that the child is dead. They look for her. Unconsciously, they are always waiting for her to appear. They don't know how to fill up their time now that they no longer have to go to the hospital everyday. They remain in their empty home, feeling that life has lost all meaning. The drugs sitting in the medicine cabinet continue to haunt them. *When should I give her a pill?* They are pills with no purpose. They should be thrown out immediately. *Should I get up in the middle of the night to check if she's breathing normally and to make sure that she isn't running a fever?* No, she will never have another fever. *But what can I do? My hands, my head, even my heart, having nothing more to do, nothing left to say. Everything is empty.*

Then, little by little, the parents become angry. The same parents who showed nothing but generosity and tenderness when their child was ill, now experience an irrational anger, and it is directed against everything and everybody. "What makes other parents so special? What have they done to deserve being spared?"

And they come to envy other parents. They ask them to account for themselves. They can't bear to look at a pregnant woman. They begrudge her the promise of life that they themselves once knew, only to be betrayed. "Where are all our friends, our parents, and all those who were so concerned immediately after the death of our child?"

When these same friends do show good intentions, they are accused of meddling in something that doesn't concern them. "Don't they have any respect for our privacy?" This aggression is sometimes directed at the doctor and the hospital staff:

"If only the specialist had told me the whole truth, I wouldn't have had the same attitude. You led me to believe in this miracle drug. And because of it my child suffered more, and all to no avail. And that first doctor, who didn't even believe that my daughter was ill. Perhaps if he had sent her to a specialist sooner, she wouldn't be dead now."

Parents may take it out on God, each other, or even on their other children. In the final analysis, they take it out on themselves; they blame, hate and accuse themselves. They end up believing that they are the reason their child didn't get better. "Maybe she wouldn't have died if we'd been more faithful in giving her her medicine. If only we'd been more careful in noticing the symptoms. If only we had called the doctor sooner."

It's important that we understand the actions and emotions of parents who are going through this painful phase. We must not avoid their company at this time, even though it's not always pleasant. Their anger is only temporary. Sometimes, it can last several months, and is linked to a deep sense of failure. I once asked a mother who had experienced this situation what attitude I should take towards such aggressive behaviour. She said, "If you don't know what to say or do, well, don't say anything, don't do anything. Just be there. Listen to us without contradicting us."

Parents' feelings of guilt can very naturally lead to depression. They may withdraw, feeling all alone. They feel like strangers in a world that refuses to understand them. They may become egocentric, and it all comes back to reinforce this devastating feeling of guilt. They even feel guilty about being alive when their children are not. "Oh my God, what have I done for you to have taken my son away from me? It isn't him that you should have chosen. It's me. John was so gentle, so kind. He was always so tender and loving."

It's important to notice the use of and focus on the pronoun *me*. One shouldn't read into it an expression of egoism, but rather a sign of confusion that has caused this parent to lock himself or herself away in unhealthy solitude. It is so difficult to help these people because, in their opinion, nobody can understand them except those who've gone through the same experience. It is now that loneliness, the feeling of solitude, sets in. They hurt every time they enter the child's empty bedroom. Every time they see the unoccupied chair at the table, or think about the toys all packed away.

They can't get used to not hearing his voice, the noise of his games. They can't look forward to the first day of classes in the fall. Or kissing their son. They begin to dream the impossible. Some parents have claimed that once the period of emptiness was over, they felt that their children were very close to them, but that it was impossible to see or touch them. This feeling can become very intense.

Some parents miss their children to the point where they become ill. One father, unable to hold back his tears, confided in me:

"If only I could see him once again, to hear him call me 'Daddy.' If only I could touch him, just for a few seconds. I'd be content with that, I wouldn't ask for anything more."

A mother once told me, as if it was in the realm of possibility:

"My little girl has been gone for almost four months now. That's long enough. It's time she came back to me."

Only time can heal these wounds. The months pass and it is the anniversary of the child's death. The first year of mourning has been very painful. Every celebration, every season, every special event, has brought back memories, both happy and sad, of the same time last year when the child was still alive. Birthdays can open wounds that have barely healed. By now, perhaps, the parents have stopped dreaming of the impossible, that their child will one day return. They have become resigned to carrying on without their child.

This return to everyday living comes about gradually. They now have to set about rebuilding; to learn all over again how to love and how to dream. The period of mourning fades away, though they will always keep a special place in their hearts for their transient child. They should now look forward to a new beginning with confidence and peace of mind.

The stages that I've just described obviously vary from one case to another. Among men, for example, the period of mourning tends to manifest itself later, but it lasts longer. Men are also more likely to suffer from physical disorders as a result of their reaction to the loss; duodenal ulcers, heart problems, or angina attacks, for example. These reactions can also vary according to the circumstances of the death. A sudden death, as the result of an accident, can create a violent but much shorter reaction. A death that follows a long illness can be accepted more easily, but it will have a longer-lasting negative effect on the parents. The degree of suffering the child has known can also bring back painful memories.

One should not underestimate the impact of the death on the child's brothers and sisters. It should be remembered that they are also touched by the illness and death of their sibling and friend. Their reactions are less evident and, more often than not, they are late in surfacing. Very often, the siblings have been unconsciously neglected by their parents, who have been so preoccupied with their sick child. The other children can be just as demanding in their need for love and affection, and they don't always take kindly to being excluded. This difficult experience can create trauma for them, which leads to unexplained fears and disturbing questions about death, often a long time after the death itself.

There is, for example, an eight-year-old who was four when his brother died. At the time, he was told that when one died one went to heaven. Today that explanation is no longer sufficient. He wants to know what happened to his brother after he died. What happens when somebody is buried? Can he die of the same illness? Does death hurt? One should always reply honestly to these questions, bearing in mind the child's age and stage of intellectual development. Remember, more than anything else, these questions represent a need for security. Children are always in need of love and understanding. To lose a child is to suffer a loss that seems impossible to overcome. Yet life continues to prove that this is not the case. I once asked a mother who had been in mourning for a year what she wanted the most. She replied, "I know that I'm perhaps asking too much, too soon. But all I really want is to be happy again."

twelve

A CHILD LIKE ANY OTHER

You are a child marked by fate,
and we forget
that you are a child like any other.
Full of dreams,
you throw body and soul
into the whirlpool of life.
At home in a world of play,
wonder and laughter
are your constant companions.
Kissed by the breath of spring
you frolic in the fresh grasses.
Always ready, you slip and slide
through the fairy-tale white of winter.
You are a child poet,
for whom the world is full of wonders.
You are a child like any other.

But you have had to leave your unfinished games behind.
You compete in a humble marathon
that's not a game your friends can play.
No matter.
You will be a winner in your own time.
We will applaud,
and you will glow with pride,
forgetting the illness
that lurks in your being.

Little child, in need of so much love,
when your tired eyes
look at other children,
do you really compare yourself to them?
Has destiny determined
that you will envy those
whom we call normal
but who are so much like you?

When you lift your head,
your head without hair,
and your big eyes ask
unspoken questions,
we know what is in your heart.
And we love you.

If by chance
you can give us a sign,
trace in the air an arabesque,
magical powers will guide your hand.
And through our love,
we will understand.

Unconscious creator,
you dream with the elements
of this world,
which take you home
to your universe.
You flee from the pity that surrounds you
because, even though you hurt,
you drink deeply from the fountain of life,
you taste its fruits, you follow its dreams.
You are a child poet.
A happy child.
A child like any other.

CONCLUSION

Despite all the information on cancer that is available, it remains a hidden reality, mysterious and formidable, that many people prefer to ignore. Throughout this book I have attempted to lift the veil and throw some light on the way in which cancer affects children. At the same time, I wanted to demystify the subject. For if one wants to engage the public in a meaningful fight against cancer, one must first of all introduce people to the enemy. They have to look it in the face and evaluate all its dimensions.

I also wanted to bear witness to the extraordinary bravery and courage of the children I meet every day at Sainte-Justine. Cancer is neither a myth nor an abstraction. It invades living beings and, in my daily work, the majority of these are children. When I speak of cancer, therefore, I speak of the children who battle against a terrible illness. I've also tried to spotlight the courage that is often displayed in the gloom of a hospital room. You will also have noticed the importance I placed on the parents of cancerous children. It is with the parents that we constantly speak at the hospital. It is they who must have confidence in us every day. It is they who give our young patients their support, their love, their strength, and their souls. I wanted to pay them a very special tribute in these pages.

I have spoken of others in the book, but upon reading it, I fear that I have talked about myself, either directly or indirectly, on several occasions. I hope that you will understand, for it is inevitable that when one speaks of a subject so close to one's heart, a subject that is one's life, the word *I* must crop up once in a while. Yet I believe that I have spoken even more in the name of the medical profession; I hope that I have done so in a manner that does not detract from its merit.

It is fashionable today, as it was in the day of Molière, to criticize doctors and to question their impartiality. The medical profession has always been one that devours those who answer its call. That is as true today as it ever was, despite what you might hear to the contrary. What I've described, what I have lived, and what I see every day at Sainte-Justine, I honestly believe can be found in every branch of medicine.

In the numerous cases described in this book, I've tried to illustrate what tremendous lengths we go to in the fight against cancer. It is impossible for the state to assume the total financial burden for this. While a large part of the expenses incurred are automatically paid for by a whole raft of social measures, including medicare in Canada, there is also pure research, certain clinical procedures, and different forms of care for both the patients and the parents that are funded by private initiatives. We cannot afford to wait until governments are ready to finance every aspect of treating the sick and the needy. They would like to, but it's just not possible. For this reason, several societies like Leucan, the Lamplighters, and the Candlelighters, associations of parents of children with leukemia or cancer, among others, have been formed to support the fight against the major illnesses that afflict our society. We should never turn our backs on their fund-raising campaigns.

AFTERWORD

"One can do nothing against death, against life, and against love," sings Nana Mouskouri. Perhaps that's true. We can't for example, choose whether we will live or die when a serious illness strikes us. We can, however, adopt radically different attitudes in our approach to it. We can give up. We can accept ignoble defeat in much the same way as those who, while in good health, prefer to lead a lifestyle that will lead to an early grave. We can also take the opposite stance and, while accepting death as inevitable, make the most of our days.

For some, however, it is much easier to let their lives fade. By that I mean their fear of death becomes greater than their will to live. Their interior balance is lost. The bird that flies into a room and the black cat that crosses their path, become omens of death. Everything around them becomes carcinogenic. They want to isolate themselves from germs, a virus, or any organic substance that can produce a mutant cell that will, in turn, produce a malignant tumor. To reassure themselves, they gorge themselves on vitamins. One can't really blame them. In their fear they have become blind. Besides, the fear of death is perfectly understandable. However, if the prospect of dying of cancer can terrify a sick person, the time that remains can give that person, paradoxical as it might seem, a unique opportunity for fulfillment. In other words, accepting the inevitable can bring about a great sense of freedom.

I could give many such examples based on my own experiences. There is a film, however, that captures everything I'm trying to say. It's called *Sunshine* and is the story of Lyn Helton, a woman suffering from a bone tumor that, at the time the film was made, was considered incurable. Instead of shutting herself away in a hospital and receiving treatment that she considered inhumane and most of all useless, she decided to devote all the time she had left to her only daughter, Jenny. She spent endless hours playing with her two-year-old daughter. The child, of course, was too young to understand the reasons behind the attention she was receiving. At the end of the film, the young woman leaves her daughter a unique heirloom; a cassette on which she explains her joys, her fears, and how she has tried to overcome those fears; a cassette on which she gives precious advice to her little girl. In this way, the young woman who was destined never to see her child grow up, cheated death. She did so by leaving her child her voice, her presence. Totally absorbed by this extension of herself, she succeeded in transforming the remaining months into an all-consuming task through which she shared with her daughter a tenderness and intimacy beyond compare. The title of the film refers to the beautiful treasure that Lyn leaves her daughter.

But make no mistake. Such a scenario doesn't only happen in the movies. I've witnessed many similar scenes over the years. Each of us has a great will to survive. We'd like to think that the admirable human machine was created to survive at least eight decades. We feel cheated if this is not the case. Unfortunately, life does not always live up to these expectations. Mother Nature has a mind of her own. She is capricious. She can change our destinies. Sometimes, it is man's own folly that adds a tragic dimension to the unforseeable. For these reasons, children, perhaps our own, can become victims of an accident, sickness, a natural disaster or even of war. Should we rebel, or bow our heads in submission? The real, and perhaps the only answer, is to accept life as it is—both the good and the bad that it entails—and to attempt to make it better.

Let us take inspiration from the Bedouin who, sitting on a sand dune, understands his life in a context where everything speaks of eternity. He knows instinctively that he will never have the time to count all the stars in the sky, or to eat all the succulent dates that hang in clusters from palm trees at the oasis. He knows that after he is gone, others will admire the exquisite desert flowers, and discover, in their turn, the rich legacy of a civilization that is four thousand years old.

Instead of complaining about the limits of his existence, he is content simply to live and to enjoy his universe of sand and silence without worrying about what cannot be. Let us follow his example and live each day to the fullest without tormenting ourselves as to whether death is waiting for us around the next bend. Live and look at life. In our fast-moving world, that is a challenge in itself. Life seems so short in our hectic society that we are often afraid to reach out and grasp it for fear of being deceived. We live fast and we live poorly. We no longer hear the singing of the birds or the chirping of crickets. Instead, we let ourselves be drugged and seduced by television advertising that would have us believe that real joy consists of lifting a glass of beer and singing its praises. Looking at life would appear to be very simple, but the opposite is true. For we shoot animals when we need neither the skin nor the meat. We wipe out acres of forest without giving a thought to the flora and fauna that are destroyed in the process. It seems that every time we have a choice to make between killing and letting live, we choose killing. Have we, in fact, lost all respect for life?

Admittedly, we are all governed by the same laws that apply to other living things. We must kill to ensure our own survival. An excellent example of this maxim exists within our very bodies. Our blood contains white cells, the majority of which belong to the family known as granulocytes. We can liken them to soldiers charged with defending our body against all bacterial aggressors. Usually, they are constantly on the move, like sentries on duty. They patrol the centre of the blood vessels. Suddenly they come face to face with an invading microbe that must be repelled. They charge the enemy, enveloping it like an amoeba and devouring it. There are no medals or citations for the brave soldiers. Having fulfilled their duty by destroying the enemy, their only reward is death. They will be succeeded by other granulocytes that, like their predecessors, will be charged with the same duty and will share the same reward.

I would like to write of other marvels hidden away inside our bodies. For it has always seemed ironic that while we have walked on the moon, we are almost totally ignorant of what goes on in our own bodies. We should touch the wall of a heart and feel the incredible elasticity there. We should attend a concert in the inner ear and watch all the small cells vibrating like the strings of a harp, set in motion by the small bones of the middle ear. We should understand the transfer of an optical image from the retina to the brain. We should watch this extraordinary computer assembling thousands of image particles to reproduce an exact copy, moving and in living colour. This miracle repeats itself almost endlessly.

Be that as it may, there's no escaping the fact that the survival of our organism, as proven to us by the granulocytes, is dependent upon this duel between life and death. There can be no life without death in one form or another. That is a universal law for all living things. Whether we like it or not, we must learn to accept the reality and inevitability of death, for it is an integral part of our daily lives. We must learn to accept the battle against death when it approaches.

Understanding that death is a given in our lives can perhaps help us not to view it as a stranger when sickness strikes. Knowing that it goes hand in hand with life will enable us to tame it more easily.

Our entire battle against cancer is waged in light of this perspective. On the one hand, we are fighting without respite a merciless enemy. On the other we are maintaining the calm conviction that death is an integral part of life.

GLOSSARY

Adenocarcinoma: any one of a large group of malignant, epithelial cell tumors of the glands.

Aklylating agent: a substance that promotes alkylation (bonding of the two helixes of DNA); this mechanism will destroy the cell when it attempts to multiply.

ALL: an abbreviation for Acute Lymphoblastic Leukemia.

AML: an abbreviation for Acute Myelogenous Leukemia.

ANLL: an abbreviation for Acute Non-Lymphoblastic Leukemia.

Alopecia: the partial or complete lack of hair resulting from normal aging, endocrine disorders, drug reactions, anti-cancer medication, or skin disease.

Analgesic: a drug that relieves pain.

Anemia: a deficiency of either hemoglobin or red blood cells.

Blood Count: the number of cells per cubic millimeter of blood; performed for a variety of diagnostic purposes.

Bone Marrow: the spongy material that fills the inner cavities of the bones; this bone marrow produces all the cellular elements of the blood.

Bone Marrow Aspiration: the removal of a small amount of bone marrow; this is done by suction with a syringe inserted usually in the hip bone or the sternum.

Cachexia: a state of malnutrition, emaciation, and debility.

Cancer: a neoplasm characterized by the uncontrolled growth of abnormal cells that tend to invade surrounding tissues and to metastasize to distant body sites.

Carcinogenic: a substance that causes cancer.

Carcinoma: a malignant epithelial neoplasm (see adenocarcinoma).

CAT-SCAN: Computerized Axial Tomography Scan (in radiology); a technique in which an EMI scanner, comprising an x-ray tube, two scintillation detectors, a line printer, teletyper, and a computer and magnetic disc unit, is used to attain a series of detailed pictures of the tissues of any part of the body. The procedure is painless, non-invasive and requires no special preparation.

Chemotherapy: treatment by chemical substances having a specific effect on the tumor cells.

Corticosteroids: any one of the natural or the synthetic hormones produced by the supra-renal gland.

Cortisone: one of the corticosteroids.

Cryosurgery or cryotherapy: a treatment using extreme cold to destroy tissue.

Diagnosis: identification of a disease or condition by a scientific evaluation of physical signs, symptoms, history, laboratory tests, and procedures.

Dyspneic: to be short of breath; labored or difficult breathing.

Ecchymosis: bruise.

Embryonic: relating to an early stage of fetal formation.

Endocrine system: the network of ductless glands and other structures that elaborate and secrete hormones directly into the blood stream.

Epithelium: the covering of the internal and the external organs of the body, including the lining of vessels, e.g., skin.

Erythrocytes: one of the formed elements in peripheral blood, containing hemoglobin and transporting oxygen.

Exocrine: of or pertaining to the process of secreting outwardly through a duct to the surface of an organ or tissue or into a vessel.

Granulocyte: one of a group of leukocytes (white blood cells) characterized by the presence of cytoplasmic granules. Their main function is to fight bacteria.

Graft-vs-Host Reaction: a reaction that may develop following bone-marrow transplants. The donor's lymphocytes are invading tissues of the recipient. Symptoms may include skin rash, blisters, diarrhea, liver dysfunction, etc.

Hematologist: a specialist in the study of blood.

Hemorrhage: the escape of blood from a ruptured vessel.

Hemoglobin: the oxygen-carrying pigment of the blood.

Hyperthermia: a higher-than-normal body temperature.

Hypothermia: a lower-than-normal body temperature.

Injection: the act of forcing a liquid into the body by means of a syringe. IV, intravenously; IM, intramuscularly; IT, into the cerebral fluid; SC, sub-cutaneously.

Intra Cranial: within the skull.

Leucocyte: a white blood cell, one of the formed elements of the circulating blood system; there are different types of leucocytes: granulocytes, lymphocytes, and monocytes.

Lymph System: a complex network of capillaries that circulate fluids from tissues to the heart.

Lymphocyte: a type of white blood cell formed in the lymph glands, spleen, thymus, and bone marrow; they produce antibodies.

Lymphoblast: a lymphocyte that is in an early stage of development.

Lymphosarcoma: a general term applied to malignant neoplastic disorders of lymphoid tissues, but not including Hodgkin's disease.

Malignant: also called virulent; tending to become worse and causing death.

Meningitis: inflammation of the membranes covering the brain and spinal cord.

Meningeal Leukemia: invasion of the cerebral and spinal fluids by leukemic cells.

Mesoderm: an intermediate layer of cells that form all types of connective tissue, bone marrow, etc.; the middle of the three cell layers of the developing embryo. It lies between the ectoderm and the endoderm. Bone, connective tissue, muscle, blood, vascular and lymphatic tissue, and the pleurae of pericardium and peritoneum are all derived from the mesoderm.

Metastasis: the process by which tumor cells spread to distant parts of the body.

Myeloblastic Leukemia: see AML.

Neoplastic Disease: another term for a malignant tumor.

Neurologist: a physician who specializes in the nervous system and its disorders.

Neuroradiology: the branch of radiology concerned with looking at the skull and the spine.

Neutrophil: a polymorphonuclear granular leucocyte (see granulocyte).

Oncogenic Virus: a virus that is able to cause a neoplastic disease.

Oncologist: a physician who specializes in the study and treatment of neoplastic diseases, particularly cancer.

Osteosarcoma: a malignant tumor arising from bone tissues.

Palliative Treatment: therapy designed to relieve or reduce the intensity of uncomfortable symptoms, but not to produce a cure.

Pancytopenia: an abnormal condition characterized by a marked reduction in the number of all of the cellular elements of the blood (red cells, white cells, and platelets).

Petechiae: tiny purple or red spots that appear on the skin as a result of minute hemorrhages within the dermal or submucosal layers.

Phagocyte: a cell that is able to surround, engulf and digest microorganisms and cellular debris.

Platelet: the smallest of the cells in the blood. Platelets are disc-shaped and contain no hemoglobin. They are essential for the coagulation of blood. Normally between 150,000 and 350,000 platelets are found in 1 cubic millimeter of blood.

Pulmonologist: a person who studies the lungs.

Radiotherapy: (radiation therapy) the treatment of neoplastic disease by using X-rays or gamma rays.

Relapse: a recurrence of the disease.

Remission: the partial or complete disappearance of the clinical and subjective characteristics of a malignant or a chronic disease.

Renal: of or pertaining to the kidney.

Reticulo Endothelial System: a functional, rather than anatomical system of the body involved primarily in defense against infection and in the disposal of the products of the breakdown of cells. It is made up of macrophages mainly present in the lungs, bone marrow, spleen, and lymph nodes.

Sarcoma: a malignant neoplasm of the soft tissues arising in fibrous, fatty, muscular, synovial, vascular, or renal tissues.

Septicemia: a systemic infection in which pathogens are present in the circulating blood stream, having spread from an infection in any part of the body.

Spinal Tap: (lumbar puncture) procedure that removes small amounts of the cerebral spinal fluid that bathes the brain and spinal cord.

Stomatitis: any inflammatory condition of the mouth.

Teratoma: a tumor composed of different kinds of tissue, none of which normally occur together or at the site of the tumor. Teratomas are most common in the ovaries, testes, and sacrococcyx area.

Thrombocytopenia: low platelet counts or absence or penuria of platelets in the blood stream.

Trophoblast: a layer of tissue that forms the wall of the blastocyte or placental mammals in the early stages of embryonic development.

Tumor: a growth of tissue characterized by progressive, uncontrolled proliferation of cells; the tumor may be localized or invasive, benign or malignant.

Tumefaction: a swelling, puffiness.

Vesicule: a tiny blister containing clear fluids.

White Blood Cells: see leucocytes.

X-ray: also called Roentgen ray. Electromagnetic radiation of shorter wavelength than visible light. X-rays can penetrate most substances and are used to investigate the integrity of certain structures or to destroy diseased tissue.

BIBLIOGRAPHY

Adams, D.W., and E.J. Deveau. *Coping With Childhood Cancer. Where Do We Go From Here?* Reston Publishing Co., 1984.

Altman, A.J. and A.D. Schwartz. *Malignant Diseases of Infancy, Childhood and Adolescence.* W.B. Saunders Co., 1983.

Antony, S. *The Discovery of Death in Childhood and After.* Basic Books Inc., 1971.

Baker, L.S. *You and Leukemia.* W.B. Saunders Co., 1978.

Bernard, J. *L'enfant, le sang et l'espoir.* Buchet/Chastel, 1984.

Bonica, J.J. and V. Ventafridda. *Advances in Pain Research and Therapy.* Raven Press, 1979.

Bureau, G. *Mona, A Mother's Story.* Clark-Irwin, 1981.

Feifel, H. *New Meanings of Death.* McGraw-Hill Co., 1977.

Kellerman, J. *Psychological Aspects of Childhood Cancer.* Charles C. Thomas Publisher, 1980.

Klein, N. *Sunshine.* Avon, 1974.

Koocher, G.P. and J.E. O'Malley. *The Damocles Syndrome: Psychological Consequences of Surviving Childhood Cancer.* McGraw-Hill Co., 1981.

Kübler-Ross, E. *Questions and Answers on Death and Dying.* New York: Macmillan, 1974.

Kübler-Ross, E. *On Children and Death.* New York: Macmillan, 1983.

Levine, A.S. *Cancer in the Young.* Masson Publishing, 1982.

Lund, D. *Eric.* J.B. Lippincott, 1974.

Moody, R. *Life After Life.* New York: Bantam Books, 1975.

Parker, M. and D. Mauger. *Children with Cancer. A Handbook for Families and Helpers.* Cassel, 1979.

Pockedly, C. *Pediatric Cancer Therapy.* Baltimore: University Park Press, 1979.

Pomminville, L. and J. Demers. *Pomme Recounts the Story of Cancer. A Big Storm in the Garden of Your Life.* Leucan, 1984.

Raimbault, G. *L'enfant et la mort.* Privat "Educateurs," 1975.

Schiff, H.S. *The Bereaved Parent.* New York: Crown Publishers, 1977.

Schweisguth, O. *Tumeurs solides de l'enfant.* Flammarion Médecine-Sciences, 1979.

Simonton, P.C. and S. Simonton. *Getting Well Again: A Self-Guide to Overcoming Cancer.* New York: Bantam Books, 1980.

Sutow, W.W. *Malignant Solid Tumors in Children: A Review.* Raven Press, 1981.

Sutow, W.W., D.J. Fernback and T.J. Vietti. *Clinical Pediatric Oncology.* C.V. Mosby Co., 1984.

Van Eys, J. and M.P. Sullivan. *Status of Curability of Childhood Cancer.* Raven Press, 1980.

Willoughby, M. and S.E. Siegel. *Hematology and Oncology (Pediatrics 1).* Butterworth Scientific, 1982.

ARTICLES

Bérubé, T. "Terry Fox—A Gift to Last." *Canadian Medical Association Journal,* 125 (1981), 284.

Clark, R.L. "Cancer 1980: Acheivements, Challengers, and Prospects." *Cancer,* 49 (1982), 1739–45.

D'Angio, G.J. "Pediatric Cancer in Perspective: Cure is Not Enough." *Cancer,* 35, 3 (1975), 866–70

D'Angio, G.J., H.W. Clatworthy, A.E. Evans, W.A. Newton and M. Tefft. "Is the Risk of Morbidity and Rate Mortality Worth the Cure?" *Cancer,* 41 (1978), 377–80.

Davidson, T. "The Bravest Children in the World." *Family Circle,* 21 July (1981), 21.

Demers, J. and H. Salvador. "La Participation des parents au traitement de l'enfant leucémique ou cancéreux." *Union médicale du Canada,* 108, 11 (1979), 1392–93.

Fiore, N. "Fighting Cancer: One Patient's Perspective." *New England Journal of Medicine,* 300, 6 (1979), 284–89.

Gale, R.P. "Medical Progress: Advances in the Treatment of Acute Myelogenous Leukemia." *New England Journal of Medicine,* 300, 21 (1979), 1189–98.

Greenberg, D.M. "The Case Against Laetrile. The Fraudulent Cancer Remedy." *Cancer,* 45 (1980), 799–807.

Hersh, E.M, E.J. Freireich, E. Frei III, and D. Hammond. "Myron R. Karon: A Tribute." *Cancer Research,* 35 (1975), 2220–21.

Karon, M. "The Physician and the Adolescent with Cancer." *Pediatric Clinics of North America,* 20, 4 (1973), 965–73.

Lansky, S.B., N.U. Cains, et al. "Childhood Cancer: Non-Medical Costs of the Illness." *Cancer,* 43 (1979), 403–08.

Lewin, R. "New Reports of a Human Leukemia Virus." *Science,* 214, (1981), 530–31.

Li, F.P. "Follow-up of Survivors of Childhood Cancer." *Cancer,* 39, 4 (1977), 1776–78.

Mauer, A.M., J.V. Simone and C.B. Pratt. "Current Progress in the Treatment of The Child with Cancer." *Journal of Pediatrics,* 91 (1977), 523–39.

Melzack, R., B.M. Mount and J.M. Gordon. "The Brompton Mixture Versus Morphine Solution Given Orally: Effect on Pain." *Canadian Medical Association Journal,* 120 (1979), 435–38.

Miller, D.R. "Childhood Acute Leukemia." *Curr. Ther.,* 28 (1981), 309–18.

Pinkel, D. "Treatment of Acute Lymphocytic Leukemia." *Cancer,* 43, 3 (1979), 1128–37.

Raimbault, G. "Children Talk about Death." *Acta Pediatric Scandinavia,* 70 (1981), 179–82.

Rivard, G.E., R.L. Momparler, J. Demers, P. Benoit, R. Raymon, K.T. Lin and L. Momparler. "Phase I Study on 5-AZA-2'-Deoxycytidine in Children with Actue Leukemia." *Leukemia Research,* 5, 6 (1981), 453–62.

Thomas, E.D. "The Role of Marrow Transplantation in the Eradication of Malignant Disease." *Cancer,* 49 (1982), 1963–68.

Siegel, S.E. "The Current Outlook for Childhood Cancer: The Medical Background," in *Psychological Aspects of Children's Cancer,* ed. by J. Kellerman. Springfield: C.E. Thomas, 1978, pp. 5–13.

Spinetta, J.J., D. Rigler and M. Karon. "Anxiety in the Dying Child." *Pediarics,* 52 (1973), 841–45.

Vernick, J. and M. Karon. "Who's Afraid of Death on a Leukemia Ward?" *American Journal of Disease of Children,* 109 (1965), 393–97.

CHILDHOOD CANCERS

TYPE	ORIGIN	SUBGROUPS
Cerebral tumors	brain	astrocytoma; medulloblastoma; ependymoma
Leukemia	bone marrow	acute and chronic A. lymphoblastic, (ALL); A. non-lymphoblastic, (ANLL, AML)
Lymphoma	lymph nodes	Hodgkin's lymphoma; Non-Hodgkin's lymphoma
Wilms' tumor (nephroblastoma)	kidney	—
Neuroblastoma	neurogenic tissue	neuroblastoma; ganglioneuroblastoma
Rhabdomyosarcoma	striated muscle	embryonal; alveolar; pleomorphic
Osteosarcoma (osteogenic sarcoma)	bone	—
Ewing's sarcoma	bone	skeletal; extra-skeletal

Retinoblastoma	retina	—
Teratoma	different kinds of tissue	yolk sac tumor; terato carcinoma
Hepatoma	liver	hepatoblastoma; hepatocarcinoma
Synoviosarcoma	synovial mem- branes	—
Chondrosarcoma	cartilaginous cells	—
Fibrosarcoma	fibrous connective tissue	—
Malignant histio- cytoma	fibroblast or histiocytes	—
Angiosarcoma	endothelial cells (vascular tissue)	—
Leiomyosarcoma	smooth muscle	—
Liposarcoma	fatty cells	—
Hemangio- pericytoma	cells surrounding blood vessels	—